Alcohol and Drug Misuse

T0258258

Alcohol and Drug Misuse

A Cochrane Handbook

Iosief Abraha MD

Regional Health Authority of Umbria
Perugia
Italy

Cristina Cusi MD

Outpatient Services – Neurology
Clinical Institutes of Specialisation
Milan
Italy

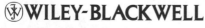

WILEY-BLACKWELL

A John Wiley & Sons, Ltd., Publication

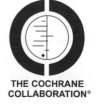

**THE COCHRANE
COLLABORATION®**

This edition first published 2012, © 2012 by John Wiley & Sons, Ltd.

This Work is a co-publication between The Cochrane Collaboration and Wiley-Blackwell. Wiley-Blackwell is an imprint of John Wiley & Sons, formed by the merger of Wiley's global Scientific, Technical and Medical business with Blackwell Publishing.

Registered office: John Wiley & Sons, Ltd, The Atrium, Southern Gate, Chichester, West Sussex, PO19 8SQ, UK

Editorial offices: 9600 Garsington Road, Oxford, OX4 2DQ, UK
111 River Street, Hoboken, NJ 07030-5774, USA

For details of our global editorial offices, for customer services and for information about how to apply for permission to reuse the copyright material in this book please see our website at www.wiley.com/wiley-blackwell.

The right of the author to be identified as the author of this work has been asserted in accordance with the UK Copyright, Designs and Patents Act 1988.

All rights reserved. No part of this publication may be reproduced, stored in a retrieval system, or transmitted, in any form or by any means, electronic, mechanical, photocopying, recording or otherwise, except as permitted by the UK Copyright, Designs and Patents Act 1988, without the prior permission of the publisher.

Designations used by companies to distinguish their products are often claimed as trademarks. All brand names and product names used in this book are trade names, service marks, trademarks or registered trademarks of their respective owners. The publisher is not associated with any product or vendor mentioned in this book. This publication is designed to provide accurate and authoritative information in regard to the subject matter covered. It is sold on the understanding that the publisher is not engaged in rendering professional services. If professional advice or other expert assistance is required, the services of a competent professional should be sought.

Library of Congress Cataloging-in-Publication Data

Abraha, Iosief.
  Alcohol and drug misuse / Iosief Abraha, Cristina Cusi.
      p. ; cm. – (Cochrane handbook)
  Includes bibliographical references and index.
  ISBN 978-0-470-65969-4 (pbk.)
    I. Cusi, Cristina.   II. Cochrane Collaboration.   III. Title.   IV. Series: Cochrane book series.
  [DNLM: 1. Substance-Related Disorders–therapy–Review.   2. Comparative Effectiveness Research–Review.   3. Early Medical Intervention–Review.   4. Social Support–Review.   WM 270]

  616.86'06–dc23

                                                                        2012020172

A catalogue record for this book is available from the British Library.

Wiley also publishes its books in a variety of electronic formats. Some content that appears in print may not be available in electronic books

Set in 9.5/12pt Minion by Toppan Best-set Premedia Limited
Printed and bound in Malaysia by Vivar Printing Sdn Bhd

1   2012

Contents

Part 2: Drugs

Psychosocial interventions

Cocaine dependence

Opioid dependence

Other drugs

Foreword

Alcohol and substance use disorders contribute directly to disability and premature deaths, and are associated with social and economic complications. Unlike in other settings, health interventions involved in substance use disorders are organised today into structured systems that require a complex approach and the involvement of professionals of different backgrounds, including primary care physicians, psychologists, neurologists and people involved in social services and education. The primary objective of this interweaving system is to enable effective interventions that are supported by scientific evidence and focused on prevention, treatment and harm reduction, while using available resources efficiently.

Epidemiological studies report that substance use is linked to specific lifestyles, and cultural and socioeconomic factors. Hence an effective prevention based on scientific evidence – such as the promotion of healthy lifestyles or the understanding of motivational processes in adolescents that permit their propensity to drink or use drugs – should be at the forefront of the strategies to reduce the burden of drug addiction.

The health system called upon for treatment has, over time, widened the object of its attention from the specific problem of 'addiction' to include the complex needs of drug users, characterised by the extreme variability of individual conditions and contexts. Therefore, a multidisciplinary therapeutic approach, integrating different types of treatment objectives, and a constant monitoring of the therapy with attention to general quality of life are required.

An improved understanding of the neurobiological basis of the reward, craving, withdrawal and relapse phases of addiction has led to promising pharmacological treatments. A range of prospects that include a combination of socio-educational and psychotherapeutic interventions also exist.

Within this context, Cochrane Systematic Reviews are a valuable source of valid evidence that identify, appraise and synthesise all the available evidence on a specific topic.

The *Cochrane Handbook of Alcohol and Drug Misuse* provides a quick overview of 59 Cochrane Systematic Reviews covering a wide range of pharmacological and psychosocial treatments for opioid, alcohol, cocaine and other substance abuse disorders. Each review is analysed here in a structured format starting with a review question, a brief background and a summary answer, followed by the results which are presented in a comprehensive and concise way. The analysis goes on to illustrate the value that the review adds to the current knowledge, the main methodological limitations of the included studies and finally the implications of the review's conclusions for future research.

The Handbook is the synthesis of the results of years of work by authors and researchers from around the globe; in this spirit of collaboration, they have earned this well-deserved acknowledgement.

Angela Bravi
Regional Health Authority of Umbria
Mental Health and Substance Abuse

Preface

The preparation and production of a Cochrane Systematic Review comprise a very long, time-consuming process, starting with a peer-reviewed publication of a protocol. To identify studies that are to be included in a review – there are often several – authors need to screen hundreds if not thousands of abstracts of published studies identified through searching electronic databases. For studies that are not indexed in these databases, individual searches are required, calling for trained personnel to trawl through journals, reports, editorials, correspondence, meeting minutes, abstracts and supplements. Once studies have been selected for inclusion, reviewers need to assure the quality of each included study before providing quantitative results, giving conclusions and submitting the results to further peer review. This enormous process of collating evidence from thousands of dedicated people around the world is made possible within the Cochrane Collaboration with its focus on the need for healthcare decision making to be based on high-quality, up-to-date research evidence.

The Cochrane Collaboration is organised in a network of different Cochrane Review Groups that have the task of preparing and maintaining Systematic Reviews on a particular healthcare sector or type of problem. Cochrane Fields are entities that embrace and facilitate the work of Review Groups and, amongst their other tasks, summarise Cochrane Reviews within the Field's scope and disseminate these summaries to stakeholders.

The Cochrane Neurological Field works predominantly with the following Cochrane Review Groups: Dementia and Cognitive Improvement; Depression, Anxiety and Neurosis; Developmental, Psychosocial and Learning Problems; Drugs and Alcohol; Epilepsy; Movement Disorders; Multiple Sclerosis; Neuromuscular Diseases; Neuro-Oncology; Stroke; Back; Incontinence; Injuries; Pain and Palliative and Supportive Care.

This *Cochrane Handbook of Alcohol and Drug Misuse* focuses on the effect of interventions on adults and adolescents who are affected by alcohol or drug addiction. It is one of a series of initiatives by the Cochrane Neurological Field to deliver and disseminate summaries of Cochrane Systematic Reviews. We trust readers will find it a helpful contribution to their clinical decision making.

Iosief Abraha and Cristina Cusi
The Cochrane Neurological Field, Italy

Acknowledgements

We acknowledge the authors of the original Systematic Reviews for their kind and generous comments and suggestions. The summaries are prepared by ourselves, but the intellectual property of the reviews belongs to the respective authors.

We acknowledge the commitment and editing support of Kathryn Mahan and the suggestions and comments received from Teresa Cantisani and Maria Grazia Celani. We also very much wish to thank Mary Banks for her efforts in making the production of the Handbook a concrete reality.

Chapter 1 **Effectiveness of brief alcohol interventions in primary care populations**[1]

Review question: Do brief interventions, delivered in general practice or based in primary care, reduce alcohol consumption in hazardous drinking?

What is known of this topic: Excessive drinking contributes significantly to social problems, physical and psychological illness, injury and death. Hidden effects include increased levels of violence, accidents and suicide.

One way to reduce consumption levels in a community may be to offer a brief intervention in primary care provided by healthcare workers such as general physicians, nurses or psychologists. The intervention offered includes providing feedback on alcohol use and harms, identifying high-risk situations for drinking and coping strategies, increasing motivation and facilitating the development of a personal plan to reduce drinking. It takes place within the time frame of a standard consultation, 5–15 minutes for a general physician, longer for a nurse.

Summary: Brief interventions appear to lower alcohol consumption generally in men. The lack of evidence of any difference in outcomes between efficacy and effectiveness trials suggests that the current literature is relevant to routine primary care. Future trials should focus on women and on delineating the most effective components of interventions.

Last assessment date: 14 February 2007

Objectives: To assess the effectiveness of brief intervention, general practice and emergency care-based primary care, to reduce alcohol consumption. To assess whether outcomes differ between trials in research settings and those in routine clinical settings. *Primary outcomes*: Self- or other reports of drinking (quantity and frequency), levels of laboratory markers and alcohol-related harm to the drinkers or to affected others. *Other outcomes*: Patient satisfaction measures and health-related quality of life.

Study population: Patients who are routinely presenting to primary care for a range of health problems and whose alcohol consumption is identified as being excessive or who have experienced harm as a result of their drinking behaviour.

Alcohol and Drug Misuse: A Cochrane Handbook, First Edition. Iosief Abraha and Cristina Cusi.
© 2012 John Wiley & Sons, Ltd. Published 2012 by John Wiley & Sons, Ltd.

Search strategy: The Cochrane Drug and Alcohol Group's Specialised Register, MEDLINE, EMBASE, CINAHL, PsycINFO, Science Citation Index, Social Science Citation Index (February 2006), Alcohol and Alcohol Problems Science Database (1972–2003) and reference lists of articles.

Results: Twenty-two randomised trials with 7619 participants were included.

After follow-up of 1 year or longer, brief intervention had lower alcohol consumption than the control group (weight mean difference: -38 grams/week (95% CI: -54 to -23); heterogeneity between trials: $I^2 = 57\%$).

Subgroup analysis (eight studies with 2307 participants) confirmed the benefit of brief intervention in men (mean difference: -57 grams/week (95% CI: -89 to -25), $I^2 = 56\%$), but not in women (mean difference: -10 grams/week (95% CI: -48 to 29). $I^2 = 45\%$). Meta-regression showed little evidence of a greater reduction in alcohol consumption with longer treatment exposure or among trials which were less clinically representative.

Extended intervention was associated with a non-significantly greater reduction in alcohol consumption than brief intervention (mean difference: -28, 95% CI: -62 to 6 grams/week, $I^2 = 0\%$).

What this review adds to the current knowledge: Pooled analyses from a significant number of studies document that brief alcohol intervention in primary care contexts results in significant reductions in weekly consumption for men, with an average drop of about six standard drinks per week in patients compared to controls. The review showed no significant reduction in alcohol consumption for women; although this may be partly due to low statistical power (as trials reporting outcomes from women enrolled only 499 participants), brief interventions for women are not yet justified.

Main limitations: A moderate level of heterogeneity. Another most likely source of bias is loss to follow-up, which was about 27% overall and significantly higher in the brief intervention arm than in the control arm (difference in rates of 3%, 95% CI: 1% to 6%).

The future: There is a clear need for more evaluative research on brief interventions with women, younger people and those from cultural minority groups. However, given the large number of trials of brief alcohol intervention showing a positive impact in men, there is no need for more of the same before such interventions are delivered in primary care. Longer treatment appeared to have little effect in significantly improving outcomes. Moreover, there is some suggestion that screening alone may result in alcohol consumption reduction, and this should be investigated further. Finally, future research directions should focus on implementation issues including a more precise specification of brief intervention components.

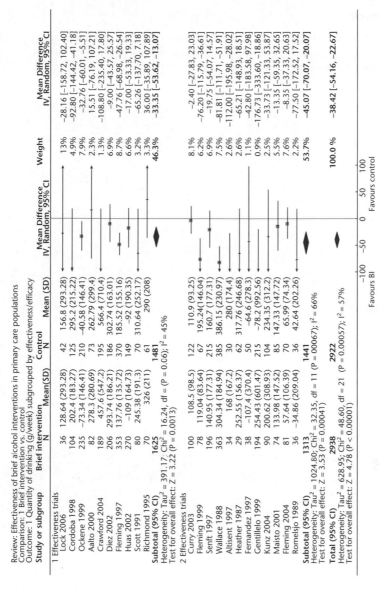

Figure 1.1 Brief intervention versus control, outcome: quantity of drinking (g/week) subgrouped by effectiveness and efficacy. Reproduced from Kaner EF, Beyer F, Dickinson HO, et al. Effectiveness of brief alcohol interventions in primary care populations. Cochrane Database Syst Rev. 2007(2):CD004148, with permission from John Wiley & Sons Ltd. Copyright © 2007 The Cochrane Collaboration.

Reference

1 Kaner EF, Beyer F, Dickinson HO, *et al.* Effectiveness of brief alcohol interventions in primary care populations. Cochrane Database Syst Rev. 2007(2):CD004148. Epub 2007/04/20.

Chapter 2 Brief interventions for heavy alcohol users admitted to general hospital wards[1]

Review question: Are brief interventions effective to reduce alcohol consumption and to improve outcomes for heavy alcohol users admitted to general hospital inpatient units?

What is known of this topic: Research suggests that a high number of patients admitted to general hospitals experience alcohol-related problems, often unrelated to the conditions they were admitted to treat.

Admission to hospital as an inpatient, in general medical wards and trauma centres, provides an opportunity whereby heavy alcohol users are accessible, have time for an intervention and may be made aware of any links between their hospitalisation and alcohol. Traditionally, interventions are offered only when individuals were diagnosed as alcohol dependent, though recent evidence has suggested benefits from intervening earlier using screening and brief interventions. Brief interventions involve a time-limited intervention that focuses on changing behaviour.

Summary: Brief interventions to heavy alcohol users admitted to general hospital wards are beneficial in terms of reduction in alcohol consumption and death rates. However, these findings are based on studies involving mainly male participants.

Last assessment date: 16 May 2011

Objectives: To determine whether brief interventions reduce alcohol consumption and improve outcomes for heavy alcohol users admitted to general hospital inpatient units. *Primary outcomes*: Alcohol consumption. *Secondary outcomes*: Hospital re-admission rates, mortality rates, alcohol-related injuries, quality of life, reduction in adverse legal events and reduction in need for institutional care.

Study population: Adults (16 years or older) admitted to a general hospital for any reason other than alcohol treatment, consuming alcohol above the

Alcohol and Drug Misuse: A Cochrane Handbook, First Edition. Iosief Abraha and Cristina Cusi.
© 2012 John Wiley & Sons, Ltd. Published 2012 by John Wiley & Sons, Ltd.

recommended safe weekly or daily amounts for the country in which the study took place.

Search strategy: The Cochrane Drug and Alcohol Group Register of Trials, Cochrane Central Register of Controlled Trials, MEDLINE, CINAHL and EMBASE (June 2008). Hand searched relevant journals, conference proceedings and contacts with experts in the field.

Results: In 11 randomised trials and controlled clinical trials, 2441 participants were identified as heavy drinkers in hospitals.

A meta-analysis of two studies showed that participants receiving brief interventions drank significantly less alcohol per week than those in the control groups at 1 year (SMD −0.18 (95% CI −0.33 to −0.03); P = 0.02), but no significant difference was observed at 6-month follow-up.

There were significantly fewer deaths in the groups receiving brief interventions than in the control group at 6 months, RR 0.42 (95% CI 0.19–0.94) and 1-year follow-up, RR 0.60 (95% CI 0.40–0.91).

No significant differences were observed between the brief intervention and control groups for other outcomes (at any follow-up time point): self-reports of alcohol consumption, laboratory markers, driving offences or number of binges.

What this review adds to the current knowledge: A Cochrane Review has indicated benefits from brief interventions in primary care, but the effectiveness of brief intervention in hospital inpatient environments remained unclear. A previous review of brief interventions in the general hospital setting found evidence for effectiveness to be inconclusive.[2]

The present review includes a further seven studies. Brief interventions to heavy alcohol users admitted to general hospital wards are beneficial in terms of reduction in alcohol consumption and death rates.

Main limitations: The heterogeneity of the outcome measure hindered the possibility of the pooling of the data.

The future: The effect of brief interventions for heavy alcohol users in general hospitals requires further investigation to determine the optimal content of brief intervention and treatment exposure. To facilitate meta-analysis, future research should utilise primary outcome measures such as alcohol consumption reporting in either units or grams of alcohol consumed or changes in alcohol consumption from baseline. Surveillance post-intervention should be at least 1 year.

Review: Brief interventions for heavy alcohol users admitted to general hospital wards
Comparison: 1 Brief interventions versus control
Outcome: 9 Sensitivity analysis: Death: smaller values indicate better outcome

Study or subgroup	Brief Intervention n/N	Control n/N	Risk Ratio M-H, Random, 95% CI	Weight	Risk Ratio M-H, Random, 95% CI
1 1 year follow up					
Chick 1985	1/7	2/78		3.5 %	0.50 [0.05, 5.40]
Freyer-Adam 2008	6/249	15/225		22.8 %	0.36 [0.14, 0.92]
Gentilello 1999	6/194	7/215		17.1 %	0.95 [0.32, 2.78]
Liu 2011	8/258	8/231		21.2 %	0.90 [0.34, 2.35]
Saitz 2007	5/141	6/146		14.6 %	0.86 [0.27, 2.76]
Sommers 2006	0/37	1/34		2.0 %	0.31 [0.01, 5.40]
Tsai 2009	5/190	12/199		18.8 %	0.44 [0.16, 1.22]
Subtotal (95% CI)	**1147**	**1128**		**100.0 %**	**0.61[0.39, 0.96]**

Total events: 31 (Brief Intervention), 51 (Control)
Heterogeneity: Tau^2 = 0.0; Chi^2 = 3.45, df = 6 (P = 0.75); I^2 = 0.0%
Test for overall effect: Z = 2.16 (P = 0.031)

```
        0.05   0.2    1      5    20
        Favours treatment    Favours control
```

Figure 2.1 Brief interventions versus control, outcome: death. Reproduced from McQueen J, Howe TE, Allan L, Mains D, Hardy V. Brief interventions for heavy alcohol users admitted to general hospital wards. Cochrane Database Syst Rev 2011(8): CD005191, with permission from John Wiley & Sons Ltd. Copyright © 2011 The Cochrane Collaboration.

References

1 McQueen J, Howe TE, Allan L, Mains D, Hardy V. Brief interventions for heavy alcohol users admitted to general hospital wards. Cochrane Database Syst Rev. 2011(8):CD005191. Epub 2011/08/13.

2 Emmen MJ, Schippers GM, Bleijenberg G, Wollersheim H. Effectiveness of opportunistic brief interventions for problem drinking in a general hospital setting: systematic review. BMJ. 2004;328(7435):318. Epub 2004/01/20.

Chapter 3 Alcoholics Anonymous and other 12-step programmes for alcohol dependence[1]

Review question: Are Alcoholics Anonymous or Twelve Step Facilitation programmes effective with alcohol-dependent patients compared to other psychosocial interventions?

What is known of this topic: Alcoholics Anonymous is an international organisation of recovering alcoholics that offers emotional support through self-help groups and a model of abstinence for people recovering from alcohol dependence, using a 12-step approach. Although it is the most common, Alcoholics Anonymous is not the only 12-step intervention available; there are other 12-step approaches labelled Twelve Step Facilitation.

Summary: The available experimental studies did not demonstrate the effectiveness of Alcoholics Anonymous or other 12-step approaches in reducing alcohol use and achieving abstinence compared with other treatments.

Last assessment date: 19 March 2006

Objectives: To assess the effectiveness of Alcoholics Anonymous (AA) and other Twelve Step Facilitation (TSF) programmes in reducing alcohol intake, achieving abstinence, maintaining abstinence, improving the quality of life of affected people and their families and reducing alcohol-associated accidents and health problems. *Primary outcomes:* Severity of dependence, retention, drop-out, reduction of drinking, abstinence and patients' and relatives' satisfaction.

Study population: Adults older than 18 years with alcohol dependence attending AA or other TSF programmes; studies on patients coerced to participate will be included, and results will be considered separately from those of studies with voluntary participation.

Alcohol and Drug Misuse: A Cochrane Handbook, First Edition. Iosief Abraha and Cristina Cusi.
© 2012 John Wiley & Sons, Ltd. Published 2012 by John Wiley & Sons, Ltd.

Search strategy: Specialized Register of Trials of the Cochrane Group on Drugs and Alcohol, the Cochrane Central Register of Controlled Trials (CENTRAL), MEDLINE, EMBASE, CINAHL (from 1982), PsycINFO (February 2005) and lists of references.

Results: Eight randomised trials with 3417 participants were included.

One small study that combined AA with other interventions concluded that AA may help patients to accept treatment and keep patients in treatment longer than alternative treatments.

Other studies reported similar retention rates regardless of treatment group.

Three studies compared AA, combined with other interventions, against other treatments and found few differences in the amount of drinks and percentage of drinking days. Severity of addiction and drinking consequence did not seem to be differentially influenced by TSF versus comparison treatment interventions.

What this review adds to the current knowledge: Overall, severity of addiction does not seem to be differentially influenced by the interventions from studies included in this review. TSF improved scores in drinking consequences in the same way as other comparison treatments, though regression to the mean cannot be discounted as a factor. There is no conclusive evidence from a number of different studies to show that AA helps patients to accept therapy and keeps patients in therapy any more or less than other interventions. Similarly, there was no evidence that other TSF interventions impacted the number remaining in treatment any more or less than relapse prevention treatment.

Main limitations: Heterogeneity across treatment, condition and outcome measure.

The future: Further large-scale studies comparing just one AA or TSF intervention with a control should be undertaken to test the efficacy of that intervention over longer follow-up periods. Further attention should be devoted to quality of life outcomes for patients and their families, as it is possible that a well-designed qualitative study could identify hypotheses for further research.

Reference

1 Ferri M, Amato L, Davoli M. Alcoholics Anonymous and other 12-step programmes for alcohol dependence. Cochrane Database Syst Rev. 2006;3:CD005032. Epub 2006/07/21.

Chapter 4 **Mentoring adolescents to prevent substance use disorders**[1]

Review question: Is mentoring adolescents an effective approach to prevent substance use disorders?

What is known of this topic: Substance use disorders are increasingly common among adolescents and young adults. Mentoring – defined as a supportive relationship in which one person offers support, guidance and assistance to the partner – can be a useful strategy to keep the mentee busy and involved in positive experiences. When mentees receive feedback and encouragement from positive mentors with whom they have bonded, they have less time to associate with users of alcohol and drugs, and have less need to use drugs and alcohol to alter mood or please peers.

Summary: Although few trials found mentoring to reduce the rate of initiation of substance use disorders, the ability of the interventions to be effective was limited by the low rates of commencing substance use during the intervention period in two studies.

Last assessment date: 5 March 2011

Objectives: To assess effectiveness of mentoring to prevent adolescent substance use disorders. *Primary outcomes*: Abstinence as measured by number of participants never starting to use drugs and/or alcohol; use of alcohol or drugs as measured by number of subjects who use alcohol or drugs at least once monthly; reduction in consumption of drugs and/or alcohol; not progressing in use of drugs or alcohol and not being involved in alcohol- or drug-related aggression or accidents.

Study population: Adolescents aged 13 to 18.

Search strategy: Cochrane CENTRAL, MEDLINE, EMBASE (July 2011), five other electronic and 11 Grey literature electronic databases, 10 websites, reference lists and experts in addictions and mentoring.

Alcohol and Drug Misuse: A Cochrane Handbook, First Edition. Iosief Abraha and Cristina Cusi.
© 2012 John Wiley & Sons, Ltd. Published 2012 by John Wiley & Sons, Ltd.

Results: Four randomised trials with 1194 adolescents were included. Three trials provided complete data.

Compared to no intervention, mentoring was found effective in preventing alcohol use in two studies (RR 0.71, 95% CI 0.57–0.90, P = 0.005). In the third trial, no significant differences were found. One study found significantly less use of 'illegal' drugs, one did not and one assessed only marijuana use and found no significant differences.

One study measured 'substance use' without separating alcohol and drugs, and found no difference for mentoring.

What this review adds to the current knowledge: Although few trials found mentoring to reduce the rate of initiation of substance use disorders, the ability of the interventions to be effective was limited by the low rates of commencing substance use disorders during the intervention period in two studies.

Main limitations: No trial reported enough detail to assess whether an adequate randomisation method was used or allocation was concealed.

The future: Randomised trials of high quality that assess the effectiveness of mentoring in students living outside the United States, not from minority backgrounds and not living in poverty with longer follow-up.

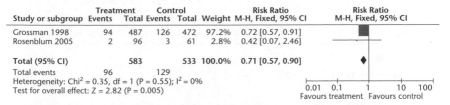

Study or subgroup	Treatment Events	Total	Control Events	Total	Weight	Risk Ratio M-H, Fixed, 95% CI	Risk Ratio M-H, Fixed, 95% CI
Grossman 1998	94	487	126	472	97.2%	0.72 [0.57, 0.91]	
Rosenblum 2005	2	96	3	61	2.8%	0.42 [0.07, 2.46]	
Total (95% CI)		583		533	100.0%	0.71 [0.57, 0.90]	
Total events	96		129				

Heterogeneity: Chi^2 = 0.35, df = 1 (P = 0.55); I^2 = 0%
Test for overall effect: Z = 2.82 (P = 0.005)

0.01 0.1 1 10 100
Favours treatment   Favours control

Figure 4.1 Mentoring versus no intervention, outcome: alcohol use in past year. Reproduced from Thomas RE, Lorenzetti D, Spragins W. Mentoring adolescents to prevent drug and alcohol use. Cochrane Database Syst Rev. 2011(11):CD007381, with permission from John Wiley & Sons Ltd. Copyright © 2011 The Cochrane Collaboration.

Reference

1 Thomas RE, Lorenzetti D, Spragins W. Mentoring adolescents to prevent drug and alcohol use. Cochrane Database Syst Rev. 2011;11:CD007381. Epub 2011/11/11.

Chapter 5 Universal school-based prevention programmes for alcohol misuse in young people[1]

Review question: Are universal school-based prevention programmes effective in preventing alcohol misuse in school-aged children up to 18 years of age?

What is known of this topic: Universal prevention strategies address the entire population within a particular setting (schools, colleges, families or communities). The aim of universal prevention is to deter or delay the onset of a disorder or problem by providing all individuals the information and skills necessary to prevent the problem. In school settings, universal prevention typically takes the form of alcohol awareness education, social and peer resistance skills, normative feedback or development of behavioural norms and positive peer affiliations.

Prevention programmes can be either specific curricula delivered as school lessons, or classroom behaviour management programmes, and can be educational, psychosocial or a combination.

Summary: Most commonly observed positive effects across programmes were for drunkenness and binge drinking. Some generic psychosocial (e.g. the Life Skills Training Programme, the Unplugged programme and the Good Behaviour Game) and developmental prevention programmes appear to be effective and could be considered as policy and practice options.

Last assessment date: 3 March 2011

Objectives: To assess the effectiveness of universal school-based prevention programmes in preventing alcohol misuse in school-aged children up to 18 years of age. *Primary outcomes*: Any direct self-reported or objective measures of alcohol consumption or problem drinking. *Other outcomes*: Alcohol initiation (age) and drunkenness initiation (age).

Study population: Children and adolescents up to 18 years attending school.

Alcohol and Drug Misuse: A Cochrane Handbook, First Edition. Iosief Abraha and Cristina Cusi.
© 2012 John Wiley & Sons, Ltd. Published 2012 by John Wiley & Sons, Ltd.

Search strategy: MEDLINE, Cochrane Central Register of Controlled Trials, EMBASE, Project CORK and PsycINFO (July 2010).

Results: Fifty-three trials were included, most of which were cluster randomised: 11 trials evaluated the effectiveness of universal school-based intervention programmes specifically focussing on the prevention of alcohol misuse in young students, and 39 trials evaluated the effectiveness of universal school-based intervention programmes with respect to the prevention of multiple factors such as misuse of alcohol, tobacco and drugs and antisocial behaviour in young students.

Data were not pooled due to heterogeneity.

Six of the 11 trials evaluating alcohol-specific interventions showed some evidence of effectiveness compared to a standard curriculum. In 14 of the 39 trials evaluating generic interventions, the programme interventions demonstrated significantly greater reductions in alcohol use through either a main or subgroup effect. Gender, baseline alcohol use and ethnicity modified the effects of interventions.

What this review adds to the current knowledge: This review identified studies that showed no effects of preventive interventions, as well as studies that demonstrated statistically significant effects. There was no easily discernible pattern in characteristics that would distinguish trials with positive results from those with no effects. Most commonly observed positive effects across programmes were for drunkenness and binge drinking. Current evidence suggests that certain generic psychosocial and developmental prevention programmes can be effective and could be considered as policy and practice options. These include the Life Skills Training Programme, the Unplugged programme and the Good Behaviour Game. A stronger focus of future research on intervention programme content and delivery context is warranted.

Main limitations: The reporting quality of trials was poor, only 3.8% of them reporting adequate method of randomisation and programme allocation concealment. Incomplete data were adequately addressed in 23% of the trials. Extensive heterogeneity across interventions, populations and outcomes.

The future: The relevance of the content and context of prevention programme delivery for programme effects is poorly understood, so studies should undertake more rigorous process evaluations alongside outcome evaluations. Reporting of programme content and context should be more detailed and systematic to enable comparison of these aspects across studies. Further improvement to study design, analysis and reporting, in line with accepted guidance, is required.

Reference

1 Foxcroft DR, Tsertsvadze A. Universal school-based prevention programmes for alcohol misuse in young people. Cochrane Database Syst Rev. 2011(5):CD009113. Epub 2011/05/13.

Chapter 6 **Universal multicomponent prevention programmes for alcohol misuse in young people**[1]

Review question: Are universal multicomponent prevention programmes effective for preventing alcohol misuse in young people?

What is known of this topic: Alcohol misuse can cause physical, psychological and social problems – in both the short term and the long term. While in school settings prevention programming typically aims to foster decision-making skills amongst young people, either through raising awareness of harms or through skill-based curricula, in family settings, parents and careers play an important role in the socialisation of young people. Universal prevention interventions seems to work when the risk factors for development of a problem are not easy to identify, are diffuse in the population and are not easily targeted by an intervention.

Summary: There is some evidence that multicomponent interventions for alcohol misuse prevention in young people can be effective. However, there is little evidence that interventions with multiple components are more effective than those with single components.

Last assessment date: 16 January 2011

Objectives: To assess the effectiveness of universal multicomponent prevention programmes in preventing alcohol misuse in school-aged children up to 18 years of age. *Primary outcomes*: Any direct self-reported or objective measures of alcohol, alcohol use, drinking more than five drinks at any one occasion and incidence of drunkenness. *Other outcomes*: Alcohol initiation (age) and drunkenness initiation (age).

Study population: Children and adolescents up to 18 years attending school.

Search strategy: MEDLINE, Cochrane Central Register of Controlled Trials, EMBASE, Project CORK and PsycINFO (July 2010).

Alcohol and Drug Misuse: A Cochrane Handbook, First Edition. Iosief Abraha and Cristina Cusi.
© 2012 John Wiley & Sons, Ltd. Published 2012 by John Wiley & Sons, Ltd.

Results: Twenty parallel-group trials were included. Data were not pooled due to important heterogeneity.

Twelve of the 20 trials showed some evidence of effectiveness compared to a control or other intervention group, with persistence of effects ranging from 3 months to 3 years.

Of the remaining eight trials, one trial reported significant effects using one-tailed tests and seven trials reported no significant effects of the multi-component interventions for reducing alcohol misuse.

Assessment of the additional benefit of multiple- versus single-component interventions was possible in seven trials with multiple arms. Only one of the seven trials clearly showed a benefit of components delivered in more than one setting.

What this review adds to the current knowledge: Results from the present review suggest that certain universal multicomponent prevention programmes can be effective and could be considered as policy and practice options. However, given the variability in effect sizes and persistence of effects between studies it is recommended that particular attention is paid to programme content and delivery context, ideally through conducting further evaluation studies alongside any further implementation in different settings. There is no clear evidence to suggest that multicomponent interventions are more effective than single-component ones.

Main limitations: The reporting quality of trials was poor, with only 25% and 5% of them reporting adequate method of randomisation and programme allocation concealment, respectively. Incomplete data were adequately addressed in about half of the trials, and this information was unclear for about 20% of the trials. Important heterogeneity across interventions, populations and outcomes.

The future: The relevance of content and context of prevention programme delivery for programme effects is poorly understood, so studies should undertake more rigorous process evaluations alongside outcome evaluations. Reporting of programme content and context should be more detailed and systematic to enable comparison of these aspects across studies. Further improvement in study sample size, design, analysis and reporting, in line with accepted guidance, is required.

Reference

1 Foxcroft DR, Tsertsvadze A. Universal multi-component prevention programmes for alcohol misuse in young people. Cochrane Database Syst Rev. 2011;9:CD009307.

Chapter 7 Universal family-based prevention programmes for alcohol misuse in young people[1]

Review Question: Are universal family-based prevention programmes effective in preventing alcohol misuse in school-aged children up to 18 years of age?

What is known of this topic: Universal prevention strategies address the entire population within a particular setting (schools, colleges, families, communities). The aim of universal prevention is to deter or delay the onset of a disorder or problem by providing all individuals the information and skills necessary to prevent the problem.

In family settings, universal prevention typically takes the form of supporting the development of parenting skills including parental support, nurturing behaviours, establishing clear boundaries or rules, and parental monitoring. Social and peer resistance skills, the development of behavioural norms and positive peer affiliations can also be addressed with a universal family-based preventive programme.

Summary: Effects of family-based prevention interventions were small but generally consistent and also persistent into the medium to longer term.

Last assessment date: 22 November 2010

Objectives: To review evidence on the effectiveness of universal family-based prevention programmes in preventing alcohol misuse in school-aged children up to 18 years of age. *Primary outcomes*: Any direct self-reported or objective measures of alcohol consumption or problem drinking. *Secondary outcomes*: Alcohol initiation, drunkenness initiation.

Study population: Children and adolescents up to 18 years attending school.

Search strategy: MEDLINE, Cochrane Central Register of Controlled Trials, EMBASE, Project CORK, and PsycINFO (2010).

Alcohol and Drug Misuse: A Cochrane Handbook, First Edition. Iosief Abraha and Cristina Cusi.
© 2012 John Wiley & Sons, Ltd. Published 2012 by John Wiley & Sons, Ltd.

Results: Twelve parallel-group trials were included. Incomplete data was adequately addressed in about half of the trials and this information was unclear for about 30% of the trials. Due to extensive heterogeneity across interventions, populations, and outcomes, the results were summarised only qualitatively.

Nine of the 12 trials showed some evidence of effectiveness compared to a control or other intervention group, with persistence of effects over the medium and longer-term. Four of these effective interventions were gender-specific, focusing on young females. One study with a small sample size showed positive effects that were not statistically significant, and two studies with larger sample sizes reported no significant effects of the family-based intervention for reducing alcohol misuse.

What this review adds to the current knowledge: Current evidence suggests that certain family-based prevention programmes can be effective and could be considered as policy and practice options. However, given variability in effect sizes and persistence of effects between studies it is recommended that particular attention is paid to programme content and delivery context, ideally through conducting further evaluation studies alongside any further implementation in different settings.

Main limitations: The reporting quality of trials was poor, only 20% of them reporting adequate method of randomisation and programme allocation concealment.

The future: The relevance of content and context of prevention programme delivery for programme effects is poorly understood, consequently studies should undertake more rigorous process evaluations alongside outcome evaluations. Reporting of programme content and context should be more detailed and systematic to enable comparison of these aspects across studies. Further improvement to study design, analysis and reporting, in line with accepted guidance is required.

Reference

1 Foxcroft DR, Tsertsvadze A. Universal family-based prevention programmes for alcohol misuse in young people. Cochrane Database Syst Rev. 2011;9:CD009308.

Chapter 8 Social norms interventions to reduce alcohol misuse in university or college students[1]

Review question: Does social norms feedback reduce alcohol misuse in university or college students?

What is known of this topic: Misuse of alcohol can result in disabilities and death. Alcohol also leads to accidents, fights and unprotected sex by young people aged 15 to 24 years. University students, when they drink, have a tendency to drink excessively. 'Social norms' refer to our perceptions and beliefs about what comprises 'normal' behaviour. People may believe that their peers drink heavily, which influences their drinking, yet much of peer influence is the result of incorrect perceptions. Normative feedback relies on the presentation of information on these misperceptions, about personal drinking profiles, risk factors and normative comparisons. Feedback can be given alone or in addition to individual or group counselling.

Summary: Web and computer feedback and individual face-to-face feedback are probably effective in reducing alcohol misuse. Significant effects were more apparent for short-term outcomes (up to 3 months). Mailed and group feedback as well as social norms marketing campaigns were not effective.

Last assessment date: 2 May 2007

Objectives: To determine whether social norms interventions reduce alcohol misuse compared with a control (assessment-only or no intervention) or other educational or psychosocial interventions in university or college students. *Primary outcomes*: Alcohol use and misuse (quantity–frequency measures), binge drinking, drinking norms and peak blood alcohol content. *Secondary outcomes*: Measures of alcohol-related problems.

Study population: Students from university or college settings.

Alcohol and Drug Misuse: A Cochrane Handbook, First Edition. Iosief Abraha and Cristina Cusi.
© 2012 John Wiley & Sons, Ltd. Published 2012 by John Wiley & Sons, Ltd.

Search strategy: The Cochrane Drugs and Alcohol Group's Register of Trials, Central, MEDLINE, EMBASE, PsycINFO and CINAHL (March 2008).

Results: Twenty-two studies with 7275 participants were included.

- *Alcohol-related problems:* Significant reduction with web and computer feedback (WF) (SMD −0.31 95% CI −0.59 to −0.02), three studies and 278 participants. No significant effect of mailed feedback (MF), individual face-to-face feedback (IFF) or group face-to-face feedback (GFF).
- *Peak blood alcohol content (BAC):* Significant reduction with WF (SMD −0.77 95% CI −1.25 to −0.28), two studies and 198 participants. No significant effect of MF or IFF.
- *Drinking frequency:* Significant reduction with WF (SMD −0.38 95% CI −0.63 to −0.13), two studies and 243 participants and with IFF (SMD −0.39 95% CI −0.66 to −0.12), two studies and 217 participants. No significant effect of MF.
- *Drinking quantity:* Significant reduction with WF (SMD −0.35 95% CI −0.51 to −0.18), five studies and 556 participants and with GFF (SMD −0.32 95% CI −0.63 to −0.02) three studies and 173 participants. No significant effect of MF or IFF.
- *Binge drinking:* Significant reduction with WF (SMD −0.47 95% CI −0.92 to −0.03), one study and 80 participants; with IFF (SMD −0.25 95% CI −0.49 to −0.02), three studies and 278 participants and with GFF (SMD −0.38 95% CI −0.62 to −0.14), four studies and 264 participants. No significant effect of MF and IFF.
- *Drinking norms:* Significant reduction with WF (SMD −0.75 95% CI −0.98 to −0.52), three studies and 312 participants.

What this review adds to the current knowledge: Individual and personalised normative interventions over the immediate and medium term appear to reduce alcohol use, misuse and related problems amongst university or college students. The use of social norms interventions should also be considered for use and study in other settings since they have the potential to be a very cost-effective intervention for reducing alcohol use and related harms. The use of new technologies, such as web- or computer-delivered interventions, could be a successful and cost-effective method for providing normative feedback. Practitioners and policy makers may wish to consider and adopt a social norms feedback approach for the prevention of alcohol misuse.

Main limitations: Only a few studies reported how important aspects of the study design were conducted, such as concealment of treatment allocation and handling of missing data. Several sources of potential bias in the individual studies were detected, for example lack of blinding of students or researchers and lack of use of self-reported outcome measures are other potential sources of bias. No direct comparisons of WF against IFF were found.

The future: Further research studies should have sound methodological quality, larger sample sizes and longer term follow-ups to provide a more thorough assessment of the effectiveness of the social norm intervention over the medium and long term. Further research is needed to test definitively the effectiveness of mailed feedback, social marketing campaigns and group feedback.

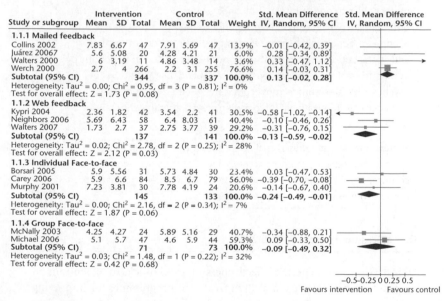

Figure 8.1 Alcohol-related problems – up to 3 months. Reproduced from Moreira MT, Smith LA, Foxcroft D. Social norms interventions to reduce alcohol misuse in university or college students. Cochrane Database Syst Rev. 2009(3):CD006748, with permission from John Wiley & Sons Ltd. Copyright © 2010 The Cochrane Collaboration.

Reference

1 Moreira MT, Smith LA, Foxcroft D. Social norms interventions to reduce alcohol misuse in university or college students. Cochrane Database Syst Rev. 2009(3): CD006748. Epub 2009/07/10.

Chapter 9 Psychosocial interventions for women enrolled in alcohol treatment during pregnancy[1]

Review question: Are psychosocial interventions in pregnant women enrolled in alcohol treatment programmes effective for improving birth and neonatal outcomes, maternal abstinence and treatment retention?

What is known of this topic: Excessive consumption of alcohol during pregnancy is associated with a wide range of adverse effects on both the mother's health and her baby's. Alcohol is associated with a continuum of birth damage which can be very serious. Pregnancy can be seen as a window of opportunity where women may seek treatment for their addictions out of concern for their unborn child and is an important point in time to treat women for their alcohol dependence. The types of psychosocial interventions most commonly used are contingency management, motivational interviewing, psychotherapy and behavioural therapy.

Summary: No randomised trials were found which fit our inclusion criteria; most trials assessed psychosocial interventions to reduce alcohol consumption in pregnant or reproductive-aged women, not pregnant or post-partum women in alcohol treatment.

Last assessment date: 15 April 2008

Objectives: To evaluate the effectiveness of psychosocial interventions in pregnant women enrolled in alcohol treatment programmes for improving birth and neonatal outcomes, maternal abstinence and treatment retention. *Primary outcomes:* Birth outcomes. *Secondary outcomes*: Abstinence outcomes and retention outcomes.

Study population: Pregnant or post-partum women in alcohol treatment programmes. No minimum level of alcohol use was required for inclusion,

Alcohol and Drug Misuse: A Cochrane Handbook, First Edition. Iosief Abraha and Cristina Cusi.
© 2012 John Wiley & Sons, Ltd. Published 2012 by John Wiley & Sons, Ltd.

no age restriction and both inpatient and outpatient treatment were included. Women receiving treatment for alcohol abuse or dependence were excluded.

Search strategy: The Cochrane Drugs and Alcohol Group's Trial Register, MEDLINE, PsycINFO, EMBASE and CINAHL (2007).

Results: The search strategy identified 958 citations. Seventeen citations were deemed relevant for full-text review, and an additional nine articles were retrieved through hand searching references, for a total of 26 articles. Following full-text review, no articles met the inclusion criteria. Data extraction and assessment of methodological quality were therefore not possible.

What this review adds to the current knowledge: Pregnancy can be seen as a window of opportunity where women may seek treatment for their addictions out of concern for their unborn child and is an important point in time to treat women for their alcohol dependence. This review sought to find all trials which compared any psychosocial intervention to other treatment or no treatment for pregnant or post-partum women in alcohol treatment.

Main limitations: No randomised trials were found which fit the inclusion criteria.

The future: Randomised trials need to be performed on pregnant alcohol-abusing women in treatment to help understand the best intervention for these women. In order to decrease the rate of foetal alcohol syndrome interventions for women with alcohol problems, those who must seek treatment comprise an important population on which to focus research.

Reference

1 Lui S, Terplan M, Smith EJ. Psychosocial interventions for women enrolled in alcohol treatment during pregnancy. Cochrane Database Syst Rev. 2008(3):CD006753. Epub 2008/07/23.

Chapter 10 **Benzodiazepines for alcohol withdrawal**[1]

Review question: Are benzodiazepines effective and safe for the management of alcohol withdrawal?

What is known of this topic: Benzodiazepines have been widely used for the treatment of alcohol withdrawal symptoms. Moreover, it is unknown whether different benzodiazepines and different regimens of administration may have the same merits.

Summary: Benzodiazepines showed a protective benefit against alcohol withdrawal symptoms, in particular seizures, when compared to placebo and a potentially protective benefit for many outcomes when compared with other drugs. Nevertheless, no definite conclusions about the effectiveness and safety of benzodiazepines were possible, because of the heterogeneity of the trials both in interventions and in the assessment of outcomes.

Last assessment date: 18 April 2010

Objectives: To evaluate the effectiveness and safety of benzodiazepines in the treatment of alcohol withdrawal. *Efficacy outcomes*: Number of subjects experiencing seizures or delirium, alcohol withdrawal symptoms, craving and global improvement of overall alcohol withdrawal. *Safety outcomes*: Number of subjects experiencing at least one adverse event and number of subjects experiencing severe, life-threatening adverse events. *Acceptability outcomes*: Additional medication needed, length of stay in intensive therapy, mortality and quality of life.

Study population: Alcohol-dependent patients diagnosed in accordance with appropriate standardised criteria (DSM-IV-R or ICD) who experienced alcohol withdrawal symptoms regardless of the severity of the withdrawal manifestations.

Alcohol and Drug Misuse: A Cochrane Handbook, First Edition. Iosief Abraha and Cristina Cusi.
© 2012 John Wiley & Sons, Ltd. Published 2012 by John Wiley & Sons, Ltd.

Search strategy: The Cochrane Drugs and Alcohol Group's Register of Trials, PubMed, EMBASE, CINAHL, EconLIT (December 2009) and searches on websites of health technology assessment and related agencies and their databases.

Results: Sixty-four studies with 4309 participants met the inclusion criteria.

- *Benzodiazepines versus placebo (three studies with 324 participants)*: Benzodiazepines performed better for seizures, RR 0.16 (95% CI 0.04–0.69). No statistically significant difference for the other outcomes considered.

- *Benzodiazepines versus other drugs (12 studies with 1228 participants)*: There was a trend in favour of benzodiazepines for seizure and delirium control, severe life-threatening side effect, drop-outs, drop-outs due to side effects and patient's global assessment score. However, no results were statistically significant. Comparing benzodiazepines versus other drugs, there is a trend in favour of benzodiazepines for seizure and delirium control, severe life-threatening side effect, drop-outs, drop-outs due to side effects and patient's global assessment score. A trend in favour of the control group was observed for CIWA-Ar scores at 48 hours and at the end of treatment. The results reach statistical significance in only one study, with 61 participants, and results on the Hamilton Anxiety Rating Scale favour control: MD −1.60 (−2.59 to −0.61).

- *Different benzodiazepines among themselves*: Results never reached statistical significance, but chlordiazepoxide performed better.

- *Fixed-schedule benzodiazepine versus symptom-triggered benzodiazepine (three studies with 262 participants)*: There was a small significant benefit of symptom-triggered regimens regarding CIWA-Ar score (change from baseline at 48 hours): MD −5.70, 95% CI −11.02 to −0.38.

- Data on safety outcomes are sparse and fragmented.

What this review adds to the current knowledge: Benzodiazepines showed a protective benefit against alcohol withdrawal symptoms, in particular seizures, when compared to placebo and a potentially protective benefit for many outcomes when compared with other drugs. Nevertheless, no definite conclusions about the effectiveness and safety of benzodiazepines were possible, because of the heterogeneity of the trials in both interventions and the assessment of outcomes.

Main limitations: Despite the considerable number of randomised trials, the large variety of outcomes and rating scales considerably limited the ability to perform a quantitative synthesis of all available data. Information on side effects was not consistently reported in the trial reports. It would be important to record more detailed data on adverse effects in these trials, since discontinuation due to side effects may affect the success of treatment. Most trials were of very small sample size, the method of randomisation was not usually described in sufficient detail, allocation concealment was frequently unclear and information on follow-up was often missing.

The future: Although a significant number of trends has emerged, most of these were small and the data for most outcomes did not reach statistical significance, indicating the need for larger, well-designed studies in this field. These studies should be limited to few, important efficacy variables such as severity of alcohol withdrawal, incidence of seizures and delirium tremens, side effects and mortality.

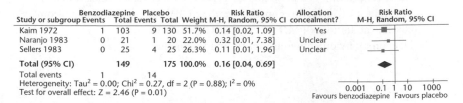

Study or subgroup	Benzodiazepine Events	Total	Placebo Events	Total	Weight	Risk Ratio M-H, Random, 95% CI	Allocation concealment?	Risk Ratio M-H, Random, 95% CI
Kaim 1972	1	103	9	130	51.7%	0.14 [0.02, 1.09]	Yes	
Naranjo 1983	0	21	1	20	22.0%	0.32 [0.01, 7.38]	Unclear	
Sellers 1983	0	25	4	25	26.3%	0.11 [0.01, 1.96]	Unclear	
Total (95% CI)		149		175	100.0%	0.16 [0.04, 0.69]		
Total events	1		14					

Heterogeneity: Tau^2 = 0.00; Chi^2 = 0.27, df = 2 (P = 0.88); I^2 = 0%
Test for overall effect: Z = 2.46 (P = 0.01)

0.001   0.1   1   10   1000
Favours benzodiazepine   Favours placebo

Figure 10.1 Benzodiazepine versus placebo, outcome: alcohol withdrawal seizures. Reproduced from Amato L, Minozzi S, Vecchi S, Davoli M. Benzodiazepines for alcohol withdrawal. Cochrane Database Syst Rev. 2010(3):CD005063, with permission from John Wiley & Sons Ltd. Copyright © 2010 The Cochrane Collaboration.

Reference

1 Amato L, Minozzi S, Vecchi S, Davoli M. Benzodiazepines for alcohol withdrawal. Cochrane Database Syst Rev. 2010(3):CD005063. Epub 2010/03/20.

Chapter 11 **Anticonvulsants for alcohol withdrawal**[1]

Review question: Are anticonvulsants effective and safe for the treatment of alcohol withdrawal?

What is known of this topic: Anticonvulsant drugs are indicated for the treatment of alcohol withdrawal, alone or in combination with benzodiazepine treatments. However, the exact role of the anticonvulsants for the treatment of alcohol withdrawal has not yet been adequately assessed.

Summary: Results of this review do not provide sufficient evidence in favour of anticonvulsants for the treatment of alcohol withdrawal.

Last assessment date: 29 December 2009

Objectives: To evaluate the effectiveness and safety of anticonvulsants in the treatment of alcohol withdrawal.

Study population: Alcohol-dependent patients diagnosed in accordance with appropriate standardised criteria (e.g., criteria of the *Diagnostic and Statistical Manual of Mental Disorders* (DSM-IV-TR) or *International Classification of Diseases* (ICD-10)).

Search strategy: The Cochrane Drugs and Alcohol Group's Register of Trials, PubMed, EMBASE, CINAHL, EconLIT (December 2009) and parallel searches on websites of health technology assessment and related agencies and their databases.

Results: Fifty-six studies, with a total of 4076 participants, met the inclusion criteria.
• *Anticonvulsants versus placebos (17 studies, six outcomes considered)*: No statistically significant differences were found for the six outcomes considered.

Alcohol and Drug Misuse: A Cochrane Handbook, First Edition. Iosief Abraha and Cristina Cusi.

© 2012 John Wiley & Sons, Ltd. Published 2012 by John Wiley & Sons, Ltd.

- *Anticonvulsants versus other drugs (32 studies, 19 outcomes considered)*: Results favour anticonvulsants only in the comparison of carbamazepine versus benzodiazepine (oxazepam and lorazepam) for alcohol withdrawal symptoms (Clinical Institute Withdrawal Assessment of Alcohol Scale – Revised (CIWA-Ar) score): three studies, 262 participants, MD −1.04 (−1.89 to −0.20). None of the other comparisons reached statistical significance.
- *Anticonvulsants plus other drugs versus other drugs (six studies, three outcomes considered)*: Results from one study with 72 participants favour paraldehyde plus chloral hydrate versus chlordiazepoxide, for the severe life-threatening side effects, RR 0.12 (0.03–0.44).
- *Different anticonvulsants between themselves (10 studies, two outcomes considered)*: No statistically significant differences for the two outcomes considered.

What this review adds to the current knowledge: Results of this review do not provide sufficient evidence in favour of anticonvulsants for the treatment of alcohol withdrawal. There are some suggestions that carbamazepine may actually be more effective in treating some aspects of alcohol withdrawal when compared to benzodiazepines, the current first-line regimen for alcohol withdrawal. Anticonvulsants seem to have limited side effects, although adverse effects are not rigorously reported in the analysed trials.

Main limitations: Most studies were of limited methodological quality, had small sample size and have been conducted in different years, and in variable populations.

The future: Further studies may change the current knowledge of this issue. Future trials should focus on important efficacy and safety measures such as the severity of the alcohol withdrawal, the incidence of seizures and delirium tremens, side effects, withdrawals and mortality.

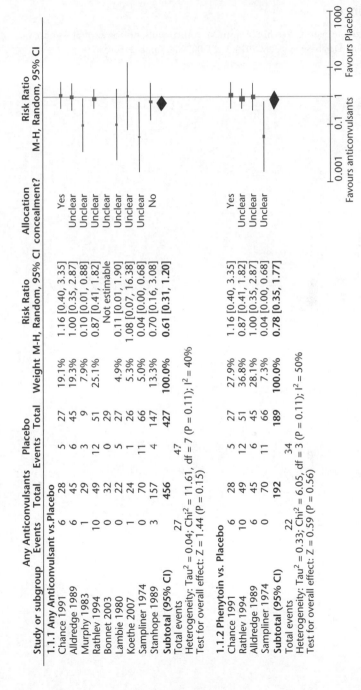

Figure 11.1 Anticonvulsant versus placebo, outcome: alcohol withdrawal seizures post treatment. Reproduced from Minozzi S, Amato L, Vecchi S, Davoli M. Anticonvulsants for alcohol withdrawal. Cochrane Database Syst Rev. 2010(3):CD005064, with permission from John Wiley & Sons Ltd. Copyright © 2010 The Cochrane Collaboration.

Reference

1 Minozzi S, Amato L, Vecchi S, Davoli M. Anticonvulsants for alcohol withdrawal. Cochrane Database Syst Rev. 2010(3):CD005064. Epub 2010/03/20.

Chapter 12 **Acamprosate for alcohol dependence**[1]

Review question: Is acamprosate effective and tolerable in comparison with placebo and other pharmacological agents in alcohol-dependent patients for supporting continuous abstinence after detoxification?

What is known of this topic: Acamprosate is a synthetic molecule with a chemical structure similar to that of the endogenous amino acid N-acetyl homotaurine. Acamprosate's precise mechanism of action is still under investigation. Current evidence suggests a multiple mediation of effects, with modulations of the N-methyl-D-aspartic acid receptor.

Summary: Acamprosate appears to be an effective and safe treatment for supporting continuous abstinence after detoxification from alcohol in dependent patients. When added to psychosocial treatment strategies, acamprosate reduced the risk of returning to any drinking after detoxification compared with placebo.

Last assessment date: 29 July 2009

Objectives: To determine the effectiveness and tolerability of acamprosate in comparison to placebo and other pharmacological agents for supporting continuous abstinence after detoxification.

Primary outcomes: Return to any drinking and cumulative abstinence duration. *Other outcomes*: Return to heavy drinking, gamma-glutamyl transpeptidase (GGT) and side effects.

Study population: Individuals with alcohol dependence according to the criteria of the *Diagnostic and Statistical Manual of Mental Disorders* (DSM-IV-TR) or *International Classification of Diseases* (ICD-10).

Search strategy: The Cochrane Drugs and Alcohol Group Specialized Register, PubMed, EMBASE and CINAHL (January 2009).

Alcohol and Drug Misuse: A Cochrane Handbook, First Edition. Iosief Abraha and Cristina Cusi.
© 2012 John Wiley & Sons, Ltd. Published 2012 by John Wiley & Sons, Ltd.

Results: Twenty-four randomised trials with 6915 participants were included.

- *Acamprosate versus placebo (24 trials):* Acamprosate was shown to significantly reduce the risk of any drinking (RR 0.86, 95% CI 0.81–0.91; heterogeneity $I^2 = 79\%$, P < 0.001); and to significantly increase the cumulative abstinence duration (WMD 10.94 (95% CI 5.08–16.81); heterogeneity $I^2 = 94\%$, P < 0.001), while secondary outcomes (GGT: seven trials, and heavy drinking: six trials) did not reach statistical significance. Diarrhoea was the only side effect that was more frequently reported under acamprosate than placebo RD 0.11 (95% CI 0.09–0.13).
- *Acamprosate versus naltrexone (three trials):* No statistically significant difference was shown: return to any drinking, RR 1.03 (95% CI 0.96–1.10); cumulative abstinence duration (WMD 2.98 (95% CI −7.45 to 13.42)) and return to heavy drinking, RR 1.04 (95% CI 0.95–1.15).

What this review adds to the current knowledge: The review confirms the effectiveness of acamprosate in alcoholism treatment. It should be noted that acamprosate was applied as an adjunctive therapy to psychosocial and psychotherapeutic interventions. Thus, strictly speaking, effect sizes rather reflect the additional benefit of adding acamprosate to psychosocial treatments than its benefit compared to placebo – a fact which often remained unconsidered in the interpretation of treatment effects.

Main limitations: As some study design features (e.g. the methods used for generating random sequences or the methods applied for allocation concealment) were omitted from trial reports, it remains unclear whether these have not been implemented or perhaps were implemented but not reported. The presence of heterogeneity should be taken into account.

The future: Further head-to-head comparisons between acamprosate and naltrexone are needed to determine the relative effectiveness of both substances and their specific profile of effectiveness.

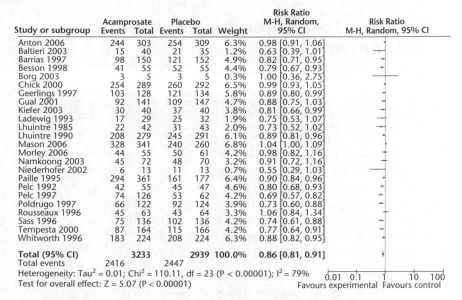

Study or subgroup	Acamprosate Events	Total	Placebo Events	Total	Weight	Risk Ratio M-H, Random, 95% CI
Anton 2006	244	303	254	309	6.3%	0.98 [0.91, 1.06]
Baltieri 2003	15	40	21	35	1.2%	0.63 [0.39, 1.01]
Barrias 1997	98	150	121	152	4.9%	0.82 [0.71, 0.95]
Besson 1998	41	55	52	55	4.4%	0.79 [0.67, 0.93]
Borg 2003	3	5	3	5	0.3%	1.00 [0.36, 2.75]
Chick 2000	254	289	260	292	6.5%	0.99 [0.93, 1.05]
Geerlings 1997	103	128	121	134	5.8%	0.89 [0.80, 0.99]
Gual 2001	92	141	109	147	4.7%	0.88 [0.75, 1.03]
Kiefer 2003	30	40	37	40	3.8%	0.81 [0.66, 0.99]
Ladewig 1993	17	29	25	32	1.9%	0.75 [0.53, 1.07]
Lhuintre 1985	22	42	31	43	2.0%	0.73 [0.52, 1.02]
Lhuintre 1990	208	279	245	291	6.1%	0.89 [0.81, 0.96]
Mason 2006	328	341	240	260	6.8%	1.04 [1.00, 1.09]
Morley 2006	44	55	50	61	4.2%	0.98 [0.82, 1.16]
Namkoong 2003	45	72	48	70	3.2%	0.91 [0.72, 1.16]
Niederhofer 2002	6	13	11	13	0.7%	0.55 [0.29, 1.03]
Paille 1995	294	361	161	177	6.4%	0.90 [0.84, 0.96]
Pelc 1992	42	55	45	47	4.6%	0.80 [0.68, 0.93]
Pelc 1997	74	126	53	62	4.2%	0.69 [0.57, 0.82]
Poldrugo 1997	66	122	92	124	3.9%	0.73 [0.60, 0.88]
Rousseaux 1996	45	63	43	64	3.3%	1.06 [0.84, 1.34]
Sass 1996	75	136	102	136	4.2%	0.74 [0.61, 0.88]
Tempesta 2000	87	164	115	166	4.2%	0.77 [0.64, 0.91]
Whitworth 1996	183	224	208	224	6.3%	0.88 [0.82, 0.95]
Total (95% CI)		**3233**		**2939**	**100.0%**	**0.86 [0.81, 0.91]**
Total events	2416		2447			

Heterogeneity: Tau^2 = 0.01; Chi^2 = 110.11, df = 23 (P < 0.00001); I^2 = 79%
Test for overall effect: Z = 5.07 (P < 0.00001)

0.01 0.1 1 10 100
Favours experimental Favours control

Figure 12.1 Acamprosate vs placebo, outcome: return to any drinking. Reproduced from Rösner S, Hackl-Herrwerth A, Leucht S, Lehert P, Vecchi S, Soyka M. Acamprosate for alcohol dependence. Cochrane Database Syst Rev. 2010(9):CD004332, with permission from John Wiley & Sons Ltd. Copyright © 2010 The Cochrane Collaboration.

Reference

1 Rosner S, Hackl-Herrwerth A, Leucht S, Lehert P, Vecchi S, Soyka M. Acamprosate for alcohol dependence. Cochrane Database Syst Rev. 2010(9):CD004332. Epub 2010/09/09.

Chapter 13 **Baclofen for alcohol withdrawal**[1]

Review question: Is baclofen effective and safe for patients with alcohol withdrawal syndrome?

What is known of this topic: Baclofen is a stereoselective gamma-aminobutyric acid B (GABAB) receptor agonist with an approved indication to control spasticity. In recent years, baclofen demonstrated its ability to suppress alcohol withdrawal signs in animal models. Baclofen produces its effect via modulating the GABAB receptor, similar to the drug gamma-hydroxybutyrate, which also has the same mechanism of action and similar effects.

Summary: The evidence of recommending baclofen for alcohol withdrawal is insufficient. More well-designed randomised trials are demanded to further prove its efficacy and safety.

Last assessment date: 5 December 2010

Objectives: To assess the efficacy and safety of baclofen for patients with alcohol withdrawal. *Efficacy outcomes*: Alcohol withdrawal seizures and delirium, alcohol withdrawal measured by the Clinical Institute Withdrawal Assessment of Alcohol Scale – Revised (CIWA-Ar) and global improvement of overall alcohol withdrawal. *Safety outcomes*: Adverse events and drop-out.

Study population: Alcohol-dependent patients diagnosed in accordance with *Diagnostic and Statistical Manual of Mental Disorders* (DSM-IV-TR) criteria for alcohol withdrawal, between 18 and 75 years of age and agreeing to abstain from alcohol for the duration of the study.

Search strategy: Cochrane Central Register of Controlled Trials, MEDLINE, EMBASE, CINAHL (from 1982 to September 2010) and other registers of on-going trials (e.g. Clinicaltrials.gov, Controlled-trials.com and EUDRACT).

Alcohol and Drug Misuse: A Cochrane Handbook, First Edition. Iosief Abraha and Cristina Cusi.
© 2012 John Wiley & Sons, Ltd. Published 2012 by John Wiley & Sons, Ltd.

Results: Only one study with 37 participants met the inclusion criteria. Baclofen oral doses of 30 mg/day in three daily administrations for 10 days, versus diazepam doses of 0.5–0.75 mg/kg in six daily administrations for 10 days, can significantly decrease the CIWA-Ar, sweating, tremors, anxiety and agitation score. Although it is slightly slower than diazepam with higher scores on days 2 and 3, on subsequent days the efficacy of baclofen and diazepam is comparable. No side effects were reported by baclofen-treated patients. On discontinuation of treatment, no withdrawal symptoms or side effects were observed.

What this review adds to the current knowledge: Only one study with a small sample size was found. Although baclofen resulted better than diazepam for several of the outcomes considered, evidence is limited to recommend baclofen in daily clinical practice.

Main limitations: The sample size of the included study was too small with only 37 participants. Allocation concealment of the included study was unknown.

The future: More well-designed randomised trials are needed. The participants should meet DSM-IV-TR criteria for alcohol withdrawal and agree to abstain from alcohol for the duration of the study. A CIWA-Ar score is a recommended scale to measure alcohol withdrawal.

Reference

1 Liu J, Wang L. Baclofen for alcohol withdrawal. Cochrane Database Syst Rev. 2011(1):CD008502. Epub 2011/01/21.

Chapter 14 Gamma-hydroxybutyrate for treatment of alcohol withdrawal and prevention of relapse[1]

Review question: Is gamma-hydroxybutyric acid (GHB) effective and safe for treatment of symptoms associated with alcohol withdrawal, and for prevention of relapses for alcohol-dependent people?

What is known of this topic: Gamma-hydroxybutyric acid is a short-chain fatty acid, a metabolite of gamma-amino-butyric acid. Its neuropharmacological and neurophysiological effects include the modulation of some neurotransmitters such as dopamine, serotonin, acetylcholine and opioids. Its alcohol-mimicking effects represent a rationale for using GHB in alcohol dependence treatment and in craving.

When it became widely available in the United States as a health food and body-building supplement during the 1980s, reports of adverse events increased to the point that the US Food and Drug Administration (FDA) ordered its removal from the market in 1990. These adverse effects range from mild hypothermia to dizziness, nausea, vomiting, weakness, loss of peripheral vision, confusion, agitation, hallucination, decreased respiratory effort, unconsciousness and coma.

Summary answer: This review does not provide evidence in favour of or against GHB compared to benzodiazepines and clomethiazole for treatment of alcohol withdrawal; but, again based on a small amount of randomised evidence, GHB appears better than naltrexone and disulfiram in maintaining abstinence and preventing craving in the medium term (3–12 months). The review does not provide evidence of a difference in side effects between GHB and benzodiazepines, naltrexone or disulfiram.

Alcohol and Drug Misuse: A Cochrane Handbook, First Edition. Iosief Abraha and Cristina Cusi.
© 2012 John Wiley & Sons, Ltd. Published 2012 by John Wiley & Sons, Ltd.

Last assessment date: 17 February 2011

Objectives: To evaluate the efficacy and safety of GHB for treatment of alcohol withdrawal and prevention of relapse. *Primary outcomes*: Drop-out rate, abstinence rate, relapse to heavy drinking and craving. *Secondary outcomes*: Length of stay in treatment, controlled drinking, number of daily drinks, number of heavy drinking days and side effects.

Study population: Alcohol-dependent patients diagnosed in accordance with appropriate standardised criteria (e.g. of the *Diagnostic and Statistical Manual of Mental Disorders* (DSM-IV-TR) or *International Classification of Diseases* (ICD-10)) or as defined by the authors.

Search strategy: The Cochrane Drugs and Alcohol Group Register of Trials, PubMed, EMBASE, CINAHL (October 2008), Econ LIT (February 2008) and reference lists of retrieved articles.

Results: Thirteen randomised trials with 648 participants were included.
* *Alcohol withdrawal syndrome*: Comparing GHB 50 mg versus placebo, results from one study (23 participants) favour GHB for withdrawal symptoms: MD −12.1 (95% CI −15.9 to −8.29), patients in the GHB group developing transitory vertigo compared to none in the placebo. In the comparison of GHB 50 mg versus clomethiazole, results from one study (21 participants) favour GHB for withdrawal symptoms: MD −3.40 (95% CI −5.09 to −1.71). GHB 100 mg versus clomethiazole results from one study (98 participants) favour clomethiazole for side effects: RR 1.84 (95% CI 1.19–2.85).
* *Abstinence rate*: At mid-term (3 or 6 months) comparing GHB 50 mg per day with placebo, one study (71 participants at 3-month follow-up) favours GHB for abstinence rate (RR 5.35, 95% CI 1.28–22.40). GHB performed better than naltrexone in two studies with 64 participants (RR 2.59, 95% CI 1.35–4.98 at 3 months) and better than disulfiram in one study with 59 participants (RR 1.66, 95% CI 0.99–2.80 at 12 months). The combination of naltrexone, GHB and escitalopram (in one study with 23 participants) was better than escitalopram alone for abstinence (RR 2.02, 95% CI 1.03–3.94 at 3 months; RR 4.58, 95% CI 1.28–16.5 at 6 months).
* *Alcohol Craving Scale*: Results favour GHB over placebo (MD −4.50, 95% CI −5.81 to −3.19 at 3 months, from one study with 71 participants) and over disulfiram at 12 months (MD −1.40, 95% CI −1.86 to −0.94, from one study with 41 participants).

What this review adds to the current knowledge: GHB is effective compared to placebo in the treatment of alcohol withdrawal, and in preventing relapses in previously detoxified alcoholics at 3 months follow-up. GHB is as effective as benzodiazepines and chlormethiazole in the treatment of alcohol withdrawal and better than naltrexone and disulfiram in maintaining abstinence. Side effects of GHB 50 mg per day are limited and manageable, and are not statistically different from those with benzodiazepines, naltrexone or disulfiram. Since abuse and toxicity are more frequent in polydrug abusers or previous abusers, GHB should be avoided in these patients.

Main limitations: Sample sizes were generally very small (range 17–98 patients). Moreover, the comparisons were varied; with GHB compared to placebo or one of several other drugs, outcomes were heterogeneous in type and timing, and recent trials studied new comparisons without retesting the previous ones.

The future: Larger trials comparing GHB to other drugs are warranted, especially because GHB is the sole drug to treat alcohol withdrawal that has also anti-craving effect.

The efficacy and safety of GHB should be evaluated in comparative trials against other drugs, whereas add-on trials are not a priority at the moment. Non-responders to GHB should be identified, and dose-finding studies are needed to understand the maximum therapeutic dose and the optimal dose schedule.

The effects of GHB for preventing alcohol withdrawal should be evaluated in unintended detoxifications that arise following major health problems, such as accidents, surgery and so on.

Review: Gamma-hydroxybutyrate (GHB) for treatment of alcohol withdrawal and prevention of relapses
Comparison: 2 GH 50 mg vs diazepam: withdrawal syndrome
Outcome: 2 CIWA-Ar score

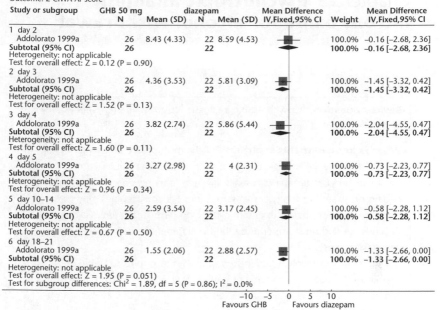

Study or subgroup	GHB 50 mg		diazepam		Mean Difference		Mean Difference
	N	Mean (SD)	N	Mean (SD)	IV,Fixed,95% CI	Weight	IV,Fixed,95% CI
1 day 2							
Addolorato 1999a	26	8.43 (4.33)	22	8.59 (4.53)		100.0%	−0.16 [−2.68, 2.36]
Subtotal (95% CI)	26		22			100.0%	−0.16 [−2.68, 2.36]
Heterogeneity: not applicable							
Test for overall effect: Z = 0.12 (P = 0.90)							
2 day 3							
Addolorato 1999a	26	4.36 (3.53)	22	5.81 (3.09)		100.0%	−1.45 [−3.32, 0.42]
Subtotal (95% CI)	26		22			100.0%	−1.45 [−3.32, 0.42]
Heterogeneity: not applicable							
Test for overall effect: Z = 1.52 (P = 0.13)							
3 day 4							
Addolorato 1999a	26	3.82 (2.74)	22	5.86 (5.44)		100.0%	−2.04 [−4.55, 0.47]
Subtotal (95% CI)	26		22			100.0%	−2.04 [−4.55, 0.47]
Heterogeneity: not applicable							
Test for overall effect: Z = 1.60 (P = 0.11)							
4 day 5							
Addolorato 1999a	26	3.27 (2.98)	22	4 (2.31)		100.0%	−0.73 [−2.23, 0.77]
Subtotal (95% CI)	26		22			100.0%	−0.73 [−2.23, 0.77]
Heterogeneity: not applicable							
Test for overall effect: Z = 0.96 (P = 0.34)							
5 day 10–14							
Addolorato 1999a	26	2.59 (3.54)	22	3.17 (2.45)		100.0%	−0.58 [−2.28, 1.12]
Subtotal (95% CI)	26		22			100.0%	−0.58 [−2.28, 1.12]
Heterogeneity: not applicable							
Test for overall effect: Z = 0.67 (P = 0.50)							
6 day 18–21							
Addolorato 1999a	26	1.55 (2.06)	22	2.88 (2.57)		100.0%	−1.33 [−2.66, 0.00]
Subtotal (95% CI)	26		22			100.0%	−1.33 [−2.66, 0.00]
Heterogeneity: not applicable							
Test for overall effect: Z = 1.95 (P = 0.051)							

Test for subgroup differences: Chi^2 = 1.89, df = 5 (P = 0.86); I^2 = 0.0%

−10 −5 0 5 10
Favours GHB   Favours diazepam

Figure 14.1 GHB versus diazepam, outcome: CIWA-Ar score. Reproduced from Leone MA, Vigna-Taglianti F, Avanzi G, Brambilla R, Faggiano F. Gamma-hydroxybutyrate (GHB) for treatment of alcohol withdrawal and prevention of relapses. Cochrane Database Syst Rev. 2010(2):CD006266, with permission from John Wiley & Sons Ltd. Copyright © 2010 The Cochrane Collaboration.

Reference

1 Leone MA, Vigna-Taglianti F, Avanzi G, Brambilla R, Faggiano F. Gamma-hydroxybutyrate (GHB) for treatment of alcohol withdrawal and prevention of relapses. Cochrane Database Syst Rev. 2010(2):CD006266.

Chapter 15 **Psychotropic analgesic nitrous oxide for alcohol withdrawal**[1]

Review question: Is psychotropic analgesic nitrous oxide (PAN) effective for treating alcohol withdrawal states?

What is known of this topic: One of the most severe consequences of alcohol dependence is the withdrawal state. The most popular current treatment is benzodiazepines, usually given in tapering doses over a period of days or titrated to the patients' symptoms. Benzodiazepines may give excessive sedation, delays in entering the long-term treatment of alcohol dependence and most importantly the development of dependence on the benzodiazepines.

PAN treatment involves administering low levels of nitrous oxide plus oxygen to the patient who remains conscious and coherent throughout gas administration. Nitrous oxide at low doses combined with a minimum of 30% oxygen differs from anaesthetic.

Summary: The review found that PAN is as effective as sedatives for managing mild to moderate alcohol withdrawal. Nevertheless, it does not provide strong evidence in favour of the benefits or harms of using PAN over sedatives in managing acute alcohol withdrawal. Further high-quality trials should be done before these findings can be confirmed.

Last assessment date: 27 December 2006

Objectives: *Primary outcomes*: Improvement of at least 50% or more from baseline of alcohol withdrawal. *Secondary outcomes*: Treatment retention and incidence of subjects entering into a rehabilitation programme.

Study population: Voluntary consenting subjects dependent on alcohol who fulfil *Diagnostic and Statistical Manual of Mental Disorders* (DSM-IV-TR)

Alcohol and Drug Misuse: A Cochrane Handbook, First Edition. Iosief Abraha and Cristina Cusi.
© 2012 John Wiley & Sons, Ltd. Published 2012 by John Wiley & Sons, Ltd.

criteria for alcohol withdrawal. Trials which include participants with alcoholic delirium were excluded.

Search strategy: Cochrane Central Register of Controlled Trials (*The Cochrane Library*, Issue 2, 2005), MEDLINE, EMBASE, CINAHL (May 2005), internet websites, reference lists of relevant articles and abstracts of the International Conferences on Alcoholism.

Results: Five studies with 212 participants were included.

PAN showed improvement of symptoms, RR 1.35 (95% CI 1.01–1.79); of the amount and duration of sedative medication and psychomotor function, WMD −8.71 (95% CI −13.71 to −3.71), and in respect to benzodiazepine. At 1 hour post intervention, no significant differences were found for depression, WMD −2.40 (95% CI −8.70 to 3.89), or anxiety, WMD −3.70 (95% CI −10.53 to 3.12).

What this review adds to the current knowledge: Results indicate that PAN may be an effective treatment of mild to moderate alcoholic withdrawal. The rapidity of the therapeutic effect of PAN therapy, coupled with the minimal sedative requirements, may enable patients to enter the psychological treatment phase more quickly than those on sedative regimens, accelerating their recovery. This review does not provide strong evidence due to the small sample sizes of the included trials.

Main limitations: Due to the difference between measured outcomes in each trial, it was not possible to conduct meta-analyses for most outcomes, and results presented from the small individual trials must be treated with caution.

The future: Further high-quality trials should be done to confirm these findings and to investigate whether the PAN therapy has fewer adverse effects than the benzodiazepines or other treatments for acute mild to moderate alcohol withdrawal states. Studies to investigate the possible cost-effectiveness of PAN by reducing costly hospital admissions and decreasing post-administration supervision also need to be performed.

42 Alcohol

Review: Psyshotropic analgesic nitrous oxide for alcoholic withdrawal states
Comparison: 1 Analgesic nitrous oxide vs. standard benzodiazepine
Outcome: 4 Positive therapeutic response

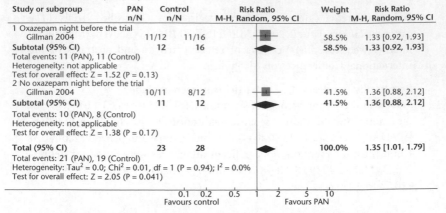

Figure 15.1 Analgesic nitrous oxide versus standard benzodiazepine, outcome: a positive therapeutic response. Reproduced from Gillman MA, Lichtigfeld FJ, Young TN. Psychotropic analgesic nitrous oxide for alcoholic withdrawal states. Cochrane Database Syst Rev. 2007(2):CD005190, with permission from John Wiley & Sons Ltd. Copyright © 2007 The Cochrane Collaboration.

Reference

1 Gillman MA, Lichtigfeld FJ, Young TN. Psychotropic analgesic nitrous oxide for alcoholic withdrawal states. Cochrane Database Syst Rev. 2007(2):CD005190. Epub 2007/04/20.

Chapter 16 **Efficacy and safety of pharmacological interventions for the treatment of alcohol withdrawal**[1]

Review question: Which pharmacological interventions are effective and safe for the treatment of alcohol withdrawal syndrome?

What is known of this topic: Alcohol dependence represents a very serious health problem worldwide with major social, interpersonal and legal interpolations. Pharmacological treatments presently used are of uncertain effectiveness, and there is even more doubt on the comparative effects and value for money.

Summary: Despite the fact that benzodiazepines showed a protective benefit against seizures, no definite conclusions were possible, because of the heterogeneity of the trials both in interventions and in the assessment of outcomes. Data on potential harms are sparse and fragmented. Results do not provide sufficient evidence in favour of anticonvulsants, baclofen or gamma-hydroxybutyric acid.

Last assessment date: 28 March 2011

Objectives: To summarise Cochrane Reviews that assess the effectiveness and safety of pharmacological interventions in the treatment of alcohol withdrawal. *Efficacy outcomes*: Alcohol withdrawal seizures, alcohol withdrawal delirium, alcohol withdrawal symptoms as measured by prespecified scales (e.g. the Clinical Institute Withdrawal Assessment of Alcohol Scale – Revised (CIWA-Ar) score) and craving. *Safety outcomes*: Adverse events, severe, life-threatening adverse events. *Acceptability outcomes*: Dropout and dropout due to adverse events.

Alcohol and Drug Misuse: A Cochrane Handbook, First Edition. Iosief Abraha and Cristina Cusi.
© 2012 John Wiley & Sons, Ltd. Published 2012 by John Wiley & Sons, Ltd.

Study population: Alcohol-dependent patients diagnosed in accordance with appropriate standardised criteria (e.g., criteria of the *Diagnostic and Statistical Manual of Mental Disorders* (DSM-IV-TR) or *International Classification of Diseases* (ICD)) who experienced alcohol withdrawal symptoms regardless of the severity of the withdrawal manifestations. All patients were included regardless of age, gender, nationality and outpatient or inpatient therapy.

Search strategy: The *Cochrane Database of Systematic Reviews* (December 2010).

Results: Five reviews, comprising 114 studies and 7333 participants, satisfied criteria for inclusion.

The outcomes considered were alcohol withdrawal seizures, adverse events and drop-outs. Comparing the five treatments with placebo, benzodiazepines performed better for seizures in three studies with 324 participants, RR 0.16 (95% CI 0.04–0.69), moderate quality of evidence. Comparing each of the five treatments versus a specific class of drugs, benzodiazepines performed better than antipsychotics for seizures in four studies with 633 participants, RR 0.24 (95% CI 0.07–0.88), high quality of evidence. Comparing different benzodiazepines and anticonvulsants among themselves in 28 comparisons, results never reached statistical significance but chlordiazepoxide performed better.

What this overview of reviews adds to the current knowledge:
Among the treatments considered, benzodiazepines showed a protective benefit against seizures when compared to placebo and a potentially protective benefit for many outcomes when compared with antipsychotics. Nevertheless, no definite conclusions about the effectiveness and safety of benzodiazepines were possible, because of the heterogeneity of the trials both in interventions and in the assessment of outcomes. Data on potential harms are sparse and fragmented. Results do not provide sufficient evidence in favour of anticonvulsants for the treatment of alcohol withdrawal, but anticonvulsants seem to have limited side effects. There is also not enough evidence of the effectiveness and safety of baclofen because only one study considered this treatment, and of gamma-hydroxybutyric acid for which no strong differences were observed in the comparisons with placebo, benzodiazepines and anticonvulsants.

Main limitations: The quality of evidence was high for 3% of the studies, moderate for 28%, low for 48% and very low for 20%. Heterogeneity and sparse data may affect the validity of the results.

The future: Most of the available evidence is of moderate quality, suggesting the need for further research. Particularly since benzodiazepines showed a potential benefit, further studies should test alternative drugs against them, and should investigate which benzodiazepine performed better for the treatment of alcohol withdrawal and the relative dose–response effect.

Reference

1 Amato L, Minozzi S, Davoli M. Efficacy and safety of pharmacological interventions for the treatment of the alcohol withdrawal syndrome. Cochrane Database Syst Rev. 2011(6):CD008537. Epub 2011/06/17.

Chapter 17 **Opioid antagonists for alcohol dependence**[1]

Review question: Are opioid antagonists effective for alcohol-dependent subjects compared to placebo or other pharmacological agents?

What is known of this topic: The treatment of alcohol dependence was exclusively dominated by psychosocial strategies for many decades. With the investigation of the neurobiological mechanism of alcohol dependence, various pharmacological agents have been examined in their potential to support alcohol-dependent patients. The glutamate antagonist acamprosate and the opioid antagonist naltrexone may block the opioid receptor system, which mediates the euphoric and pleasurable effects of alcohol. Evidence is needed to support the use of opioid antagonists to reduce the effect of alcohol dependence.

Summary: Naltrexone was more effective than placebo in reducing the amount and frequency in drinking without causing dependency.

Last assessment date: 8 October 2010

Objectives: To determine the effectiveness and tolerability of opioid antagonists in the treatment of alcohol dependence. *Primary outcomes*: Return to heavy drinking, return to any drinking and drinking days. *Secondary outcomes*: Heavy drinking days, consumed amount per drinking day, gamma-glutamyl transpeptidase and side effects.

Study population: Individuals with alcohol dependence according to the criteria of the *Diagnostic and Statistical Manual of Mental Disorders* (DSM-IV-TR) or *International Statistical Classification of Diseases* (ICD-10).

Search strategy: The Cochrane Drugs and Alcohol Group Specialized Register, PubMed, EMBASE, CINAHL (January 2010) and inquiries made to manufacturers and researchers for unpublished trials.

Results: Fifty randomised trials with 7793 patients were included.

Alcohol and Drug Misuse: A Cochrane Handbook, First Edition. Iosief Abraha and Cristina Cusi.
© 2012 John Wiley & Sons, Ltd. Published 2012 by John Wiley & Sons, Ltd.

• *Naltrexone versus placebo*: Compared to placebo, naltrexone was effective in reducing the risk of heavy drinking by 17% (40 studies, RR 0.83, 95% CI 0.76–0.90) and in decreasing the number of drinking days by about 4% (MD −3.89, 95% CI −5.75 to −2.04). Significant effects were also demonstrated for the secondary outcomes of the review including heavy drinking days (MD −3.25, 95% CI −5.51 to −0.99); consumed amount of alcohol (MD −10.83, 95% CI −19.69 to −1.97) and gamma-glutamyltransferase, (MD −10.37, 95% CI −18.99 to −1.75), while effects on return to any drinking missed statistical significance (RR 0.96, 95% CI 0.92–1.00).

Side effects of naltrexone were mainly gastrointestinal problems (e.g. nausea: RD 0.10, 95% CI 0.07–0.13) and sedative effects (e.g. daytime sleepiness: RD 0.09, 95% CI 0.05–0.14). Based on a limited study sample, effects of injectable naltrexone and nalmefene missed statistical significance.

What this review adds to the current knowledge: Naltrexone appears to be an effective and safe strategy in the treatment of alcoholism. Even though the size of treatment effects might appear moderate in their amount, these should be valued against the background of the relapsing nature of alcoholism and the limited therapeutic options currently available for its treatment.

Main limitations: The reporting of clinical trials with opioid antagonists was clear and comprehensible in most study publications. Nevertheless, as some study design features (e.g. the methods used for generating random sequences or the methods applied for allocation concealment) were omitted from trial reports, it remains unclear whether these have not been implemented or whether they were implemented but not reported. The presence of heterogeneity should be taken into account. A stricter adherence to methodological standards of reporting as outlined in the CONSORT statement would help to remove methodological remaining doubts and uncertainties. There was a moderate to high level of heterogeneity.

The future: Direct comparisons between oral versus injectable naltrexone would help to further specify the advantages and disadvantages of different forms of application.

The identification of patient characteristics which determine a patient's responsiveness to the available psychosocial and pharmacological interventions is indispensable for the deduction of elaborated techniques of combining therapeutic strategies and their tailoring to the individual treatment goals and therapeutic needs of patients.

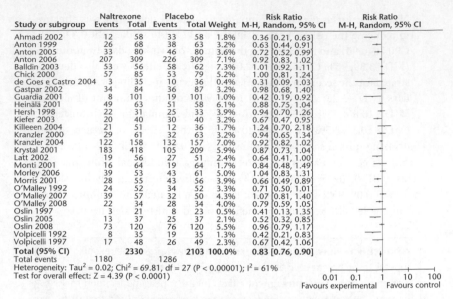

Study or subgroup	Naltrexone Events	Naltrexone Total	Placebo Events	Placebo Total	Weight	Risk Ratio M-H, Random, 95% CI
Ahmadi 2002	12	58	33	58	1.8%	0.36 [0.21, 0.63]
Anton 1999	26	68	38	63	3.2%	0.63 [0.44, 0.91]
Anton 2005	33	80	46	80	3.6%	0.72 [0.52, 0.99]
Anton 2006	207	309	226	309	7.1%	0.92 [0.83, 1.02]
Balldin 2003	53	56	58	62	7.3%	1.01 [0.92, 1.11]
Chick 2000	57	85	53	79	5.2%	1.00 [0.81, 1.24]
de Goes e Castro 2004	3	35	10	36	0.4%	0.31 [0.09, 1.03]
Gastpar 2002	34	84	36	87	3.2%	0.98 [0.68, 1.40]
Guardia 2001	8	101	19	101	1.0%	0.42 [0.19, 0.92]
Heinälä 2001	49	63	51	58	6.1%	0.88 [0.75, 1.04]
Hersh 1998	22	31	25	33	3.9%	0.94 [0.70, 1.26]
Kiefer 2003	20	40	30	40	3.2%	0.67 [0.47, 0.95]
Killeeen 2004	21	51	12	36	1.7%	1.24 [0.70, 2.18]
Kranzler 2000	29	61	32	63	3.2%	0.94 [0.65, 1.34]
Kranzler 2004	122	158	132	157	7.0%	0.92 [0.82, 1.02]
Krystal 2001	183	418	105	209	5.9%	0.87 [0.73, 1.04]
Latt 2002	19	56	27	51	2.4%	0.64 [0.41, 1.00]
Monti 2001	16	64	19	64	1.7%	0.84 [0.48, 1.49]
Morley 2006	39	53	43	61	5.0%	1.04 [0.83, 1.31]
Morris 2001	28	55	43	56	3.9%	0.66 [0.49, 0.89]
O'Malley 1992	24	52	34	52	3.3%	0.71 [0.50, 1.01]
O'Malley 2007	39	57	32	50	4.3%	1.07 [0.81, 1.40]
O'Malley 2008	22	34	28	34	4.0%	0.79 [0.59, 1.05]
Oslin 1997	3	21	8	23	0.5%	0.41 [0.13, 1.35]
Oslin 2005	13	37	25	37	2.1%	0.52 [0.32, 0.85]
Oslin 2008	73	120	76	120	5.5%	0.96 [0.79, 1.17]
Volpicelli 1992	8	35	19	35	1.3%	0.42 [0.21, 0.83]
Volpicelli 1997	17	48	26	49	2.3%	0.67 [0.42, 1.06]
Total (95% CI)		2330		2103	100.0%	0.83 [0.76, 0.90]
Total events	1180		1286			

Heterogeneity: Tau^2 = 0.02; Chi^2 = 69.81, df = 27 (P < 0.00001); I^2 = 61%
Test for overall effect: Z = 4.39 (P < 0.0001)

0.01   0.1   1   10   100
Favours experimental   Favours control

Figure 17.1 Naltrexone versus placebo, outcome: return to heavy drinking.
Reproduced from Rösner S, Hackl-Herrwerth A, Leucht S, Vecchi S, Srisurapanont M,
Soyka M. Opioid antagonists for alcohol dependence. Cochrane Database Syst Rev.
2010(12):CD001867, with permission from John Wiley & Sons Ltd. Copyright
© 2010 The Cochrane Collaboration.

Reference

1 Rösner S, Hackl-Herrwerth A, Leucht S, Vecchi S, Srisurapanont M, Soyka M.
Opioid antagonists for alcohol dependence. Cochrane Database Syst Rev. 2010
(12):CD001867.

Chapter 18 **Pharmacologic interventions for pregnant women enrolled in alcohol treatment**[1]

Review question: Which pharmacologic interventions for pregnant women enrolled in alcohol treatment programmes are effective and safe for improving birth and neonatal outcomes, maternal abstinence and treatment retention?

What is known of this topic: During pregnancy, alcohol consumption may increase the risk of miscarriage, reduce growth and impair the mental development of the baby. Different drugs are given to lessen the effects during detoxification. These include benzodiazepines, phenothiazines and chlormethiazone, used to reduce anxiety and insomnia. Anti-depressants may also be given after withdrawal. Disulfiram, naltrexone and acamprosate are used in more severe cases to decrease cravings for alcohol and maintain abstinence. A systematic review is needed to gather the evidence of which treatments are effective.

Summary: The review authors could not identify any randomised trial evaluating the effectiveness of pharmacologic interventions to improve maternal, birth and infant outcomes in pregnant women enrolled in alcohol treatment programmes.

Last assessment date: 25 March 2009

Objectives: To evaluate the effectiveness of pharmacologic interventions in pregnant women enrolled in alcohol treatment programmes for improving birth and neonatal outcomes, maternal abstinence and treatment retention. *Primary outcomes*: Birth outcomes. *Secondary outcomes*: Abstinence and retention.

Study population: Pregnant or post-partum women enrolled in alcohol treatment programmes.

Alcohol and Drug Misuse: A Cochrane Handbook, First Edition. Iosief Abraha and Cristina Cusi.
© 2012 John Wiley & Sons, Ltd. Published 2012 by John Wiley & Sons, Ltd.

Search strategy: The Cochrane Drugs and Alcohol Group's Trial Register, MEDLINE, EMBASE (August 2008), CINAHL, PsycINFO (June 2008) and reference lists of articles.

Results: The search strategy identified 793 citations. Twenty-three citations were deemed relevant for a full-text review; an additional 10 articles were retrieved through hand searching references, for a total of 33 articles. Following full-text review, no articles met the inclusion criteria. Data extraction and assessment of methodological quality were therefore not possible.

What this review adds to the current knowledge: This reviews adds only that there is no current randomised trial published in the medical literature.

Main limitations: Not applicable since no study was included.

The future: Quality epidemiologic outcome research is needed due to the magnitude of suffering that alcohol use has on the public's health. Rather than pushing future research towards randomised controlled trials (RCTs), the review authors suggest that quality cohort studies with appropriate unexposed controls to assess potential confounders such as continued maternal alcohol use and socioeconomic variables would be more appropriate and cost effective.

Reference

1 Smith EJ, Lui S, Terplan M. Pharmacologic interventions for pregnant women enrolled in alcohol treatment. Cochrane Databas Syst Rev. 2009(3):CD007361.

Chapter 19 **School-based prevention for illicit substance use disorders**[1]

Review question: Which interventions delivered in schools are effective in preventing or reducing substance use disorders among young people?

What is known of this topic: Drug addiction is a social and medical problem among adolescents and is characterised by an uncontrollable compulsion to seek drugs. Relapsing is common and interventions intended to prevent use of drugs are needed. Primary interventions should be aimed to reduce first use, or prevent the transition from experimental use to addiction. School is the appropriate setting for preventive interventions.

Summary: Programmes which develop individual social skills are the most effective form of school-level intervention for the prevention of early substance use disorders.

Last assessment date: 26 April 2005

Objectives: Evaluation of the effectiveness of school-based interventions versus usual curricular activities or a different school-based intervention. *Primary outcomes*: Drug knowledge, drug attitudes, acquirement of personal skills, peer and adult substance use disorders, intention to use drugs, use of drugs and changes in behaviours.

Study population: Primary or secondary school pupils formed the target population. Studies targeting special populations were excluded.

Search strategy: The Cochrane Drug and Alcohol Group's Trial Register (February 2004), the Cochrane Central Register of Controlled Trials (*The Cochrane Library*, Issue 2, 2004), MEDLINE (1966 to February 2004), EMBASE (1988 to February 2004), other databases and reference lists of review articles.

Results: 29 randomised trials and three controlled prospective studies were included with 46 539 participants.

Alcohol and Drug Misuse: A Cochrane Handbook, First Edition. Iosief Abraha and Cristina Cusi.
© 2012 John Wiley & Sons, Ltd. Published 2012 by John Wiley & Sons, Ltd.

Randomised trials

- *Knowledge versus usual curricula*: Knowledge-focused programmes improve drug knowledge (SMD 0.91; CI 95% 0.42–1.39).
- *Skills versus usual curricula*: Skills-based interventions increase drug knowledge (WMD 2.60; CI 95% 1.17 to 4.03), decision-making skills (SMD 0.78; CI 95% 0.46 to 1.09), self-esteem (SMD 0.22; CI 95% 0.03 to 0.40), peer pressure resistance (RR 2.05; CI 95% 1.24–3.42), drug use (RR 0.81; CI 95% 0.64–1.02), marijuana use (RR 0.82; CI 95% 0.73–0.92) and hard drug use (RR 0.45; CI 95% 0.24–0.85).
- *Skills versus knowledge*: No differences are evident.
- *Skills versus affective*: Skills-based interventions are better than affective ones only in self-efficacy (WMD 1.90; CI 95% 0.25 to 3.55).

Controlled prospective studies: Comparisons did not give statistically significant results.

What this review adds to the current knowledge: The results of this systematic review demonstrate that programmes which develop individual social skills are the most effective form of school-level intervention for the prevention of early drug use.

School-based programmes providing only information or focused only on the affective dimension, however, should be confined within the context of tightly controlled and randomised evaluations.

Main limitations: The quality of reporting was limited in many studies. Allocation concealment was not clearly reported in all trials. In eight studies, loss to follow-up ranged from 25% to 45%. Overall, 23 studies were evaluated as of moderate quality, and six as of low quality. In addition, there were very few data of sufficient validity on long-term effect of the intervention.

The future: Studies on the effect of single components when added to the basic intervention (e.g. peer influence, booster sessions and involvement of parents) have not been sufficiently investigated to allow reliable conclusions. The interaction between programmes and other social context variables also deserves attention. Authors should make efforts to reduce the number of flawed studies by preferring randomised designs, monitoring the conduction of the observation, reducing attrition, choosing a correct strategy of analysis, making their results comparable with those already published, choosing 'hard' outcomes and scales already validated and accepted and reporting all data useful for the estimation of validity: absolute numbers, relative risks and statistical indicators.

Review: School-based prevention for illicit drugs' use
Comparison: 1 knowledge versus usual curricula
Outcome: 1 drug knowledge

Study or subgroup	Treatment N	Mean (SD)	Control N	Mean (SD)	Std. Mean Difference IV, Random, 95% CI	Weight	Std. Mean Difference IV, Random, 95% CI
Corbin 1993	16	17.06 (2.86)	19	12.63 (4.57)		27.8%	1.11 [0.39, 1.83]
Jones 1995	12	17 (2.52)	8	12.5 (3.42)		16.9%	1.48 [0.45, 2.52]
Sigelman 2003	86	0.91 (0.11)	79	0.81 (0.2)		55.4%	0.62 [0.31, 0.94]
Total (95% CI)	114		106			100.0%	0.91 [0.42, 1.39]

Heterogeneity: Tau^2 = 0.08; Chi^2 = 3.55, df = 2 (P = 0.17); I^2 = 44%
Test for overall effect: Z = 3.66 (P = 0.00025)

-10 -5 0 5 10
Favours control   Favours treatment

Figure 19.1 Knowledge versus usual curricula, outcome: drug knowledge. Reproduced from Faggiano F, Vigna-Taglianti FD, Versino E, Zambon A, Borraccino A, Lemma P. School-based prevention for illicit drugs use. Cochrane Database Syst Rev. 2005(2):CD003020, with permission from John Wiley & Sons Ltd. Copyright © 2005 The Cochrane Collaboration.

Reference

1 Faggiano F, Vigna-Taglianti FD, Versino E, Zambon A, Borraccino A, Lemma P. School-based prevention for illicit drugs use. Cochrane Database Syst Rev. 2005(2):CD003020.

Chapter 20 Interventions for prevention of substance use disorders by young people delivered in non-school settings[1]

Review question: Which interventions delivered in non-school settings are effective in preventing or reducing substance use disorders among young people?

What is known of this topic: The prevalence of illicit substance use disorders is increasing among young people. Preventive interventions are required both at school and in non-school settings. Interventions in non-school settings (including youth clubs, emergency rooms, colleges, young offender institutions, the family and the community) may seek to target non-users in order to prevent the initiation of use of any drugs, existing users with a view to the minimisation of harms or both groups. Interventions may also be universal in orientation, targeting entire populations, or be directed at specific groups defined by prior substance use disorders or other risk characteristics.

Summary: Although motivational interviewing and some family interventions may have some benefit, evidence of effectiveness of the considered interventions is limited.

Last assessment date: 1 November 2005

Objectives: To summarise the current evidence about the effectiveness of interventions delivered in non-school settings intended to prevent or reduce substance use disorders by people younger than 25 years; to investigate whether interventions' effects are modified by the type and setting of the intervention and the age of young people targeted and to identify areas where more research is needed. *Outcome measures*: Substance use disorder, initiation of substance use disorder or reduction or cessation of substance use disorder, substance dependence, death, hospitalisation, treatment for drug-related health problems and criminal activity.

Study population: People younger than 25 years, either illicit drug users or non-users. Studies that included older participants were included if the

Alcohol and Drug Misuse: A Cochrane Handbook, First Edition. Iosief Abraha and Cristina Cusi.
© 2012 John Wiley & Sons, Ltd. Published 2012 by John Wiley & Sons, Ltd.

number of older participants was small and the intervention was targeted at young people, or if data were published or could be provided for young participants separately.

Search strategy: The Cochrane Central Register of Controlled Trials, MEDLINE, EMBASE, PsycINFO, SIGLE, CINAHL, ASSIA (2004) and reference lists of review articles.

Results: Seventeen studies, nine cluster randomised studies with 253 clusters and eight individually randomised studies with 1230 participants, were included.

Four types of intervention were evaluated: motivational interviewing or brief intervention, education or skills training, family interventions and multicomponent community interventions. The presence of heterogeneity and the paucity of trials hinder the possibility for firm conclusions. One study of motivational interviewing suggested that this intervention was beneficial on cannabis use. Three family interventions each, evaluated in only one study, suggested that they may be beneficial in preventing cannabis use. The studies of multicomponent community interventions did not find any strong effects on substance use disorder outcomes, and the two studies of education and skills training did not find any differences between the intervention and control groups.

What this review adds to the current knowledge: There is insufficient evidence to establish whether any of the interventions considered in this review are effective in preventing or reducing substance use disorders by young people.

Main limitations: Blinding was not possible to perform due to the type of interventions; in most trials there was a high level of loss to follow-up and allocation concealment was unclear.

The future: Future trials should have standardised outcome measures and should measure substantive substance use disorders, determine economic and health outcomes and use a sufficiently large sample size to show clinically important differences in these outcomes. When cluster randomised design is used, trials should be designed and analysed taking clustering into account.

Reference

1 Gates S, McCambridge J, Smith LA, Foxcroft DR. Interventions for prevention of drug use by young people delivered in non-school settings. Cochrane Database Syst Rev. 2006(1):CD005030.

Chapter 21 **Case management for persons with substance use disorders**[1]

Review question: Is the use of case management for people with substance use problems effective in successfully enhancing linkage with other services and reducing illicit substance use outcomes?

What is known of this topic: Subjects with alcohol and other substance use disorders (AOD) experience difficulties accessing community services, including substance use treatment. One strategy for linking patients with AOD with relevant services is case management, where a single case manager is responsible for linking patients with multiple relevant services.

Summary: Current evidence suggests that case management can enhance linkage with other services. However, evidence that case management reduces substance use or produces other beneficial outcomes is limited.

Last assessment date: 6 August 2007

Objectives: To assess whether case management reduces substance use, improves quality of life and favours the linkage of patients with community services. *Primary outcome:* Substance use, alcohol use, employment and income, physical health, legal issues, family and social relations, mental health and living situation. *Other outcomes*: Treatment participation and retention, service utilization (not including case management services), rehospitalisation and satisfaction with the intervention received.

Study population: Persons with substance use disorders (dependence on any substance). Studies including people with other mental disorders are eligible, if substance use disorders are present in the entire sample.

Search strategy: The Cochrane Controlled Trials Register, MEDLINE, EMBASE, LILACS, PsycINFO, Biological Abstracts (2000), reference searching, personal communication, conference abstracts and book chapters on case management.

Results: Fifteen studies were included.

Outcomes on illicit substance use disorders were reported from seven studies with 2391 patients. The effect size for illicit substance use disorders

---

Alcohol and Drug Misuse: A Cochrane Handbook, First Edition. Iosief Abraha and Cristina Cusi.
© 2012 John Wiley & Sons, Ltd. Published 2012 by John Wiley & Sons, Ltd.

was small and not significant (SMD 0.12, CI −0.09 to 0.29, P = 0.20). Substantial heterogeneity was found (I^2 = 69.9%).

Linkage to other treatment services was reported in 10 studies with 3132 patients. The effect size for linkage was moderate (SMD 0.42, 95% CI 0.21 to 0.62, P < 0.001), but substantial heterogeneity was found (I^2 = 85.2%).

A single, large trial of case management with two arms showed that case management was superior to psycho-education and drug counselling in reducing substance use disorders.

What this review adds to the current knowledge: Case management effectively linked people with substance use disorders to community and treatment services as compared to treatment as usual or other viable treatment options, such as psycho-education or brief interventions.

Main limitations: Substantial heterogeneity and several methodological limitations were present in the studies included.

The future: Studies that evaluate the extent of successful linkage as a mediator of other treatment outcomes (e.g. criminal involvement and substance use disorders), effective strategies for implementing case management in 'real life' and the effect of case management dosage are needed. These studies need to be of high methodological quality.

Review: Case management for persons with substance use disorders
Comparison: 1 Case Management versus treatment as usual.
Outcome: 1 Illicit drug use outcomes

Study or subgroup	Treatment N	Mean(SD)	Control N	Mean(SD)	Std. Mean Difference IV, Random, 95% CI	Weight	Std. Mean Difference IV, Random, 95% CI
Coviello 2006	71	0.1 (1)	40	0 (1)		10.4%	0.10 [−0.29, 0.49]
Martin 1993	56	−0.02 (1)	63	0 (1)		11.2%	−0.02 [−0.38, 0.34]
Morgenstern 2006	135	0.58 (1)	156	0 (1)		15.2%	0.58 [0.34, 0.81]
Rapp 1998	249	0.24 (1)	228	0 (1)		17.1%	0.24 [0.06, 0.42]
Rhodes 1997	395	0.1 (1)	734	0 (1)		18.9%	0.10 [−0.02, 0.22]
Sorensen 2003	80	0 (1)	71	0.28 (1)		12.4%	−0.28 [−0.60, 0.04]
Sorensen 2005 a	28	0.03 (1)	29	0 (1)		7.5%	0.03 [−0.49, 0.55]
Sorensen 2005 b	28	0 (1)	28	0.11 (1)		7.4%	−0.11 [−0.63, 0.42]
Total (95% CI)	**1042**		**1349**			**100.0%**	**0.12 [−0.06, 0.29]**

Heterogeneity: Tau^2 = 0.04; Chi^2 = 23.25, df = 7 (P = 0.002); I^2 = 70%
Test for overall effect: Z = 1.27 (P = 0.20)
Test for subgroup differences: Not applicable

−1   −0.5   0   0.5   1
Favours control   Favours experimental

Figure 21.1 Case management versus treatment as usual, outcome: illicit drug use outcomes. Reproduced from Hesse M, Vanderplasschen W, Rapp RC, Broekaert E, Fridell M. Case management for persons with substance use disorders. Cochrane Database Syst Rev. 2007(4):CD006265, with permission from John Wiley & Sons Ltd. Copyright © 2007 The Cochrane Collaboration.

Reference

1 Hesse M, Vanderplasschen W, Rapp RC, Broekaert E, Fridell M. Case management for persons with substance use disorders. Cochrane Database Syst Rev. 2007 (4):CD006265.

Chapter 22 **Motivational interviewing for substance use disorders**[1]

Review question: Is motivational interviewing effective for substance use disorders, retention in treatment, readiness to change and number of repeat convictions?

What is known of this topic: Motivational interviewing is a widely used client-centred, semi-directive method for enhancing intrinsic motivation to change by exploring and resolving ambivalence. However, little is known about this intervention in terms of effectiveness.

Summary: Motivational interviewing can reduce the extent of substance abuse compared to no intervention. The evidence is mostly of low quality, so further research is very likely to have an important impact on our confidence in the estimate of effect and is likely to change the estimate.

Last assessment date: 27 March 2011

Objectives: To assess the effectiveness of motivational interviewing for substance use cessation (measured by self-report, report by collaterals, urine analysis or blood samples) and reduction in substance use disorders (measured the same way). *Other outcomes*: Retention in treatment, improved motivation for change and number of repeat convictions.

Study population: Participants defined as having substance use, dependency or addiction, but not misuse.

Search strategy: The Cochrane Library, MEDLINE, EMBASE, PsycINFO (November 30, 2010), 18 other electronic databases, five websites, four mailing lists and reference lists from included studies and reviews.

Alcohol and Drug Misuse: A Cochrane Handbook, First Edition. Iosief Abraha and Cristina Cusi.
© 2012 John Wiley & Sons, Ltd. Published 2012 by John Wiley & Sons, Ltd.

Results: Fifty-nine studies with a total of 13 342 participants were included.

- *Motivational interviewing versus no treatment*: Motivational interviewing showed a significant effect on substance use which was strongest at post-intervention (SMD 0.79, 95% CI 0.48 to 1.09) and weaker at short follow-up (SMD 0.17, 95% CI 0.09 to 0.26), and medium follow-up (SMD 0.15, 95% CI 0.04 to 0.25). For long follow-up, the effect was not significant (SMD 0.06, 95% CI −0.16 to 0.28).
- *Motivational interviewing versus treatment as usual*: There were no significant differences between motivational interviewing and treatment as usual for follow-up post-intervention, short follow-up and medium follow-up. Motivational interviewing resulted better than assessment and feedback for medium follow-up (SMD 0.38, 95% CI 0.10 to 0.66). For short follow-up, there was no significant effect. For other active interventions, there were no significant effects for either follow-up.

Data were limited to make any conclusion about retention in treatment, readiness to change or repeat convictions.

What this review adds to the current knowledge: Participants who received motivational interviewing have reduced their use of substances more than those who have not received any treatment. However, it seems that other active treatments, treatment as usual and being assessed and receiving feedback can be as effective as motivational interviewing. There were not enough data to conclude about the effects of motivational interviewing on retention in treatment, readiness to change or repeat convictions.

Main limitations: Most of the trials did not report the method of allocation concealment. There is a possibility of outcome reporting bias.

The future: Further research on how motivational interviewing works is needed before performing randomised trials of low risk of bias.

Review: Motivational interviewing for substance abuse
Comparison: 1 MI versus no intervention
Outcome: 1 Extent of substance use

Study or subgroup	Control N	MI N	Std. Mean Difference (SE)	Std. Mean Difference IV, Random, 95% CI	Weight	Std. Mean Difference IV, Random, 95% CI
1 Post-intervention						
Ball 2007a	29	34	0.47 (0.26)		34.7%	0.47 [−0.04, 0.98]
Connors 2002	36	40	0.878 (0.241)		40.2%	0.88 [0.41, 1.35]
Kelly 2000	16	16	1.245 (0.386)		15.9%	1.25 [0.49, 2.00]
Stotts 2006	14	17	0.801 (0.507)		9.2%	0.80 [−0.19, 1.79]
Subtotal (95% CI)					100.0%	**0.79 [0.48, 1.09]**

Heterogeneity: Tau^2 = 0.00; Chi^2 = 3.04,
df = 3 (P = 0.39); I^2 = 1%
Test for overall effect: Z = 5.10 (P < 0.00001)

2 Short f-u						
Ball 2007	20	40	−0.028 (0.346)		1.4%	−0.03 [−0.71, 0.65]
Carey 2006	81	81	0.19 (0.111)		9.8%	0.19 [−0.03, 0.41]
Carroll 2006a	178	173	0.097 (0.076)		15.4%	0.10 [−0.05, 0.25]
Feldstein 2007	15	40	0.345 (0.305)		1.8%	0.35 [−0.25, 0.94]
Kay-Lambkin 2009	30	35	−0.048 (0.25)		2.6%	−0.05 [−0.54, 0.44]
Kelly 2000	16	16	1.23 (0.386)		1.2%	1.23 [0.47, 1.99]
MarijuanaTP 2004	148	146	0.32 (0.118)		9.0%	0.32 [0.09, 0.55]
Martin 2008	20	20	−0.099 (0.317)		1.7%	−0.10 [−0.72, 0.52]
Mastroleo 2010	82	82	0.276 (0.161)		5.6%	0.28 [−0.04, 0.59]
Morgenstern 2009	80	70	0.299 (0.162)		5.6%	0.30 [−0.02, 0.62]
Naar-King 2007	26	25	−0.041 (0.283)		2.1%	−0.04 [−0.60, 0.51]
Peterson 2006	94	92	−0.004 (0.102)		11.0%	0.00 [−0.20, 0.20]
Schaus 2009	182	181	0.25 (0.11)		10.0%	025 [0.03, 0.47]
Stein 2002	92	95	0.084 (0.103)		10.9%	0.08 [−0.12, 0.29]
Wood 2007	83	84	0.231 (0.095)		12.0%	0.23 [0.04, 0.42]
Subtotal (95% CI)					100.0%	**0.17 [0.09, 0.26]**

Heterogeneity: Tau^2 = 0.01; Chi^2 = 18.40,
df = 14 (P = 0.19); I^2 = 24%
Test for overall effect: Z = 4.08 (P = 0.000046)

3 Medium f-u						
Brown 2010	92	92	0.042 (0.148)		9.8%	0.04 [−0.25, 0.33]
Carey 2006	81	81	−0.019 (0.157)		8.9%	−0.02 [−0.33, 0.29]
Connors 2002	36	40	0.38 (0.232)		4.7%	0.38 [−0.07, 0.83]
Copeland 2001	69	78	0.525 (0.453)		1.3%	0.53 [−0.36, 1.41]
Emmen 2005	62	61	−0.2 (0.181)		7.1%	−0.20 [−0.55, 0.15]
Freyer-Adam 2008	249	225	0.064 (0.109)		15.0%	0.06 [−0.15, 0.28]
Kay-Lambkin 2009	30	35	0.424 (0.252)		4.0%	0.42 [−0.07, 0.92]
Marsden 2006	176	166	0.099 (0.108)		15.1%	0.10 [−0.11, 0.31]
Morgenstern 2009	80	70	0.37 (0.172)		7.7%	0.37 [0.03, 0.71]
Schaus 2009	182	181	0.2 (0.11)		14.8%	0.20 [−0.02, 0.42]
Stein 2009	92	95	0.173 (0.164)		8.3%	0.17 [−0.15, 0.49]
Winters 2007	27	26	0.657 (0.287)		3.2%	0.66 [0.09, 1.22]
Subtotal (95% CI)					100.0%	**0.15 [0.04, 0.25]**

Heterogeneity: Tau^2 = 0.01; Chi^2 = 14.06,
df = 11 (P = 0.23); I^2 = 22%
Test for overall effect: Z = 2.78 (P = 0.0055)

4 Long follow-up						
Schaus 2009	182	181	0.06 (0.11)		100.0%	0.06 [−0.16, 0.28]
Subtotal (95% CI)					100.0%	**0.06 [−0.16, 0.28]**

Heterogeneity: not applicable
Test for overall effect: Z = 0.55 (P = 0.59)

$$-2 \quad -1 \quad 0 \quad 1 \quad 2$$
Favours control   Favours MI

Figure 22.1 Motivational interview versus no intervention, outcome: extent of substance use. Reproduced from Smedslund G, Berg RC, Hammerstrom KT, *et al.* Motivational interviewing for substance abuse. Cochrane Database Syst Rev. 2011;5:CD008063, with permission from John Wiley & Sons Ltd. Copyright © 2011 The Cochrane Collaboration.

Reference

1 Smedslund G, Berg RC, Hammerstrom KT, *et al.* Motivational interviewing for substance abuse. Cochrane Database Syst Rev. 2011(5):CD008063.

Chapter 23 **Therapeutic communities for substance use disorders**[1]

Review question: Are therapeutic communities effective in reducing drug and alcohol dependence?

What is known of this topic: Therapeutic communities (TC) are drug-free residential settings that use a hierarchical model of care to treat people with a range of substance misuse problems. Treatment stages reflect increased levels of personal and social responsibility. Peer influence is used to help individuals learn to assimilate social norms and develop more effective social skills. In the TC approach, individuals themselves are the main contributor to the process of change.

Summary: The methodological limitations inherent to the included studies hinder any conclusion in favour of or against the efficacy of TC.

Last assessment date: 1 November 2005

Objectives: To determine the effectiveness of TC versus other treatments for substance use disorders, and to investigate whether effectiveness is modified by client or treatment characteristics. *Outcome measure*: Illicit substance use disorders, alcohol use, retention in treatment, reasons for withdrawal from treatment, Addiction Severity Index, imprisonment, employment, overdoses, substance use arrests and death due to all causes or drug related.

Study population: People who sought treatment or were ordered by the court to obtain treatment with any substance misuse or dependency problem.

Search strategy: The Cochrane Central Register of Controlled Trials (Issue 2, 2005), MEDLINE, EMBASE, PsycINFO, CINAHL and SIGLE (March 2004). Reference lists of studies were scanned.

Results: Seven studies were included.

Heterogeneity between studies precluded any pooling of data; results are summarised for each trial individually.

Alcohol and Drug Misuse: A Cochrane Handbook, First Edition. Iosief Abraha and Cristina Cusi.
© 2012 John Wiley & Sons, Ltd. Published 2012 by John Wiley & Sons, Ltd.

- *TC versus community residence*: No significant differences for treatment completion. Residential versus day TC: attrition (first 2 weeks), and abstinence rates at 6 months were significantly lower in the residential treatment group.
- *Standard TC versus enhanced abbreviated TC*: The number of employed was higher in standard TC, RR 0.78 (95% CI 0.63–0.96).
- *Three-month versus 6-month programme within modified TC, and 6-month versus 12-month programme within standard TC*: Completion rate was higher in the 3-month programme, and the retention rate (40 days) was significantly greater with the 12-month than 6-month programme.

Two trials evaluated TCs within a prison setting: one reported significantly fewer re-incarcerated 12 months after release from prison in the TC group compared with no treatment, RR 0.68 (95% CI 057–0.81). In the other trial, people treated in prison with TC compared with Mental Health Treatment Programmes showed significantly fewer re-incarcerations, RR 0.28 (95% CI 0.13–0.63); criminal activity, RR 0.69 (95% CI 0.52–0.93) and alcohol and drug offences, RR 0.62 (95% CI 0.43–0.90) 12 months after release from prison.

What this review adds to the current knowledge: Evidence of the efficacy of therapeutic communities for treatment of drug misuse and dependency is limited. Prison TC may be better than prison to prevent re-offending post release for inmates. However, methodological limitations of the studies may have introduced bias, and firm conclusions cannot be drawn due to limitations of the existing evidence.

Main limitations: Significant heterogeneity limited the possibility of pooling data. Most of the studies were of limited methodological quality. None of the trials reported the method of allocation or the blinding of the outcome evaluator. All trials were at high risk of attrition bias.

The future: Randomised trials of high quality with the aim of minimising attrition at the early stages of trial are required. In addition, outcome measures need to be standardised.

Reference

1 Smith LA, Gates S, Foxcroft D. Therapeutic communities for substance related disorder. Cochrane Database Syst Rev. 2006(1):CD005338.

Chapter 24 Interventions for drug-using offenders in the courts, secure establishments and the community[1]

Review question: Are interventions for drug-using offenders effective in reducing criminal activity and substance use disorders in the courts, secure establishments and community-based settings?

What is known of this topic: The link between substance use disorders and crime is well recognised, and drug-using offenders represent a socially excluded group who may experience problems in relation to their substance use disorders. Efforts have been made to enable people with drug problems to live healthy, crime-free lives. A number of studies and previous systematic reviews have considered the effectiveness of drug treatment interventions for drug misusers in the general population, mixed populations of offenders and non-offenders and drug treatment in a specific setting or country with limited outcome measures. This review considers interventions for drug-using offenders under the care of the criminal justice system.

Summary: Evidence about the overall effectiveness of drug treatment programmes for offenders under the care of the criminal justice system is limited.

Last assessment date: 18 May 2006

Objectives: To assess the effectiveness of interventions for drug-misusing offenders in reducing criminal activity and drug misuse across a range of criminal justice settings. *Primary outcome*: Substance use disorders and criminal activity. *Other outcomes*: Health status, information on concurrent psychiatric illness, cost and cost effectiveness.

Study population: Individuals who have been referred by the criminal justice system at baseline to the study. Offenders were in police custody, being processed by the courts system and residing in secure establishments (e.g. prisons or special hospitals) or based in the community (i.e. under the care of the probation service).

Alcohol and Drug Misuse: A Cochrane Handbook, First Edition. Iosief Abraha and Cristina Cusi.
© 2012 John Wiley & Sons, Ltd. Published 2012 by John Wiley & Sons, Ltd.

Search strategy: MEDLINE, EMBASE (October 2004), PsycINFO (January 2004), Pascal, SciSearch (Science Citation Index; November 2004) and 13 other sources.

Results: Twenty-four studies with 8936 participants were included.

No trials studied the outcome substance use disorders.

Results show that when comparing a court-based community pre-trial release with drug testing and sanctions versus routine pre-trial, for arrest at 90 days results favour the comparison group (OR 1.33, 95% CI 1.04–1.70).

Comparing therapeutic community with aftercare with a mental health programme with a waiting list control, considering incarceration at 12 months (OR 0.37, 95% CI 0.16–0.87), results favour the treatment.

Comparing intensive supervision with routine parole or probation, for recidivism (OR 1.98, 95% CI 1.01–3.87), results favour the comparison group. No statistically significant difference between the groups for arrest (OR 1.49, 95% CI 0.88–2.51); drug arrest (OR 1.10, 95% CI 0.50–2.39), conviction (OR 0.93, 95% CI 0.55–1.58) and incarceration at one year (OR 0.88, 95% CI 0.50–1.54).

Comparing intensive supervision and increased surveillance with intensive supervision alone, no statistically significant difference between the groups for recidivism (OR 2.09, 95% CI 0.86–5.07), arrest (OR 1.22, 95% CI 0.51–2.88), drug arrest (OR 1.29, 95% CI 0.35–4.85), conviction (OR 1.14, 95% CI 0.22–5.91) and incarceration (OR 1.30, 95% CI 0.39–4.30) at one year.

What this review adds to the current knowledge: Although several studies were published, limited conclusions can be drawn about the effectiveness of drug treatment programmes for drug-using offenders in the courts or the community. This is partly due to the broad range of studies and the heterogeneity of the different outcome measures presented.

Therapeutic communities with aftercare show promising results for the reduction of substance use disorders and criminal activity in drug-using offenders. Standardisation of outcome measures and costing methodology would help improve the quality of research conducted in the area.

Main limitations: Studies used different outcome measures that caused heterogeneity.

The future: Future studies with sound methodological quality with standardised outcome measures are needed.

Reference

1 Perry A, Coulton S, Glanville J, Godfrey C, Lunn J, McDougall C, *et al*. Interventions for drug-using offenders in the courts, secure establishments and the community. Cochrane Database Syst Rev. 2006(3):CD005193.

Chapter 25 Psychosocial interventions for pregnant women in outpatient illicit drug treatment programmes compared to other interventions[1]

Review question: Do psychosocial interventions translate into less illicit drug use, greater abstinence, better birth outcomes or greater clinic attendance in pregnant women?

What is known of this topic: Women using illicit drugs while pregnant are more likely to give birth early and have low-weight infants that are at risk of neonatal abstinence syndrome and requiring intensive care. The provision of psychosocial interventions for pregnant women may reduce the risk of these complications by leading them to undergo prenatal drug treatment.

There is evidence for the effectiveness of psychosocial interventions in this population; however, to our knowledge, no systematic review on the subject has been undertaken.

Summary: The present evidence suggests that contingency management strategies are effective in improving retention of pregnant women in illicit drug treatment programmes as well as in transiently reducing illicit substance use disorders. There was no evidence to support the use of motivational interviewing.

Last assessment date: 2 August 2007

Objectives: To evaluate the effectiveness of psychosocial interventions in pregnant women enrolled in illicit drug treatment programmes on birth and neonatal outcomes, on attendance and retention in treatment as well as on maternal and neonatal drug abstinence. *Obstetrical outcomes*: Birth weight, gestational age at birth and placental abruption. *Neonatal outcomes*: Neonatal abstinence syndrome, admission to and length of time spent in neonatal intensive care unit and use of primary substance use. *Other outcomes*: Retention in treatment, treatment attendance and prenatal care attendance.

Alcohol and Drug Misuse: A Cochrane Handbook, First Edition. Iosief Abraha and Cristina Cusi.
© 2012 John Wiley & Sons, Ltd. Published 2012 by John Wiley & Sons, Ltd.

Study population: Pregnant women enrolled in illicit drug treatment programmes.

Search strategy: The Cochrane Drugs and Alcohol Group's Trial Register (May 2006), the Cochrane Central Register of Trials (2005), MEDLINE, EMBASE, CINAHL (August 2006) and reference lists of articles.

Results: Nine trials involving 546 pregnant women were included. Five studies with 346 women considered contingency management (CM), and four studies with 266 women considered manual-based interventions such as motivational interviewing (MI).

The main finding was that CM led to better study retention. There was only minimal effect of CM on illicit drug abstinence. In contrast, motivational interviewing led towards poorer study retention, although this did not approach statistical significance. For both, no difference in birth or neonatal outcomes was found, but this was an outcome rarely captured in the studies.

What this review adds to the current knowledge: This systematic review found that contingency management is effective in improving retention of pregnant women in illicit drug treatment programmes but with minimal effects on their abstaining from illicit drugs. Motivational interviewing over three to six sessions may, if anything, lead to poorer retention in treatment. These findings are based on nine controlled trials over 14 days to 24 weeks, five of which used contingency management (346 women) and four of which (266 women) considered motivational interviewing.

Main limitations: The overall methodological quality was low. None of the trials adequately described any methods of allocation concealment or whether the outcomes were assessed blindly. Outcome reporting bias is another potential threat to the validity of the results.

The future: Large randomised trials of high quality with obstetrically meaningful and standardised endpoints as well as with longer follow-ups to examine whether psychosocial interventions help pregnant women with illicit substance use disorders are required. Poor obstetrical outcomes should not be an exclusion criterion to study participation, as these events are essential.

Reference

1 Terplan M, Lui S. Psychosocial interventions for pregnant women in outpatient illicit drug treatment programmes compared to other interventions. Cochrane Database Syst Rev. 2007(4):CD006037.

Chapter 26 **Psychosocial interventions for cocaine and psychostimulant amphetamine related disorders**[1]

Review question: Are psychosocial interventions effective for treating psychostimulant dependence?

What is known of this topic: Chronic consumption of cocaine and psychostimulant amphetamines results in development of stereotyped behaviour, paranoia and possibly aggressive behaviour. Psychosocial treatments for psychostimulant use disorder are supposed to improve compliance and promote abstinence.

Summary: There is little significant behavioural change with reductions in rates of drug consumption following psychosocial intervention.

Last assessment date: 20 May 2007

Objectives: To investigate the efficacy (as measured by urine samples, reported use of psychostimulants or relapse, frequency of drug intake, changes in craving for the drug and severity of dependence) and acceptability (as measured by total number of drop-outs at the end of the trial, side effects and number of drop-outs) of psychosocial interventions for treating psychostimulant dependence when compared to other psychosocial interventions, medications or no intervention. *Other outcomes*: Death, medical problems, legal problems, social and family relations, employment and support.

Study population: Participants with any diagnosis for psychostimulant use disorder, irrespective of pattern of use, gender and age.

Search strategy: Cochrane Library, EMBASE, MEDLINE, LILACS (May 2006), reference searching, personal communication, conference abstracts, unpublished trials from the pharmaceutical industry and book chapters on treatment of psychostimulant dependence.

Alcohol and Drug Misuse: A Cochrane Handbook, First Edition. Iosief Abraha and Cristina Cusi.
© 2012 John Wiley & Sons, Ltd. Published 2012 by John Wiley & Sons, Ltd.

Results: Twenty-seven randomised studies with 3663 participants were included.

The wide heterogeneity in the interventions evaluated did not allow to provide a summary estimate of effect. The most studied psychosocial intervention was the approach grounded in a cognitive-behavioural framework, particularly relapse prevention and contingency reinforcement interventions (grouped as cognitive-behavioural therapies), followed by drug counselling.

The comparisons between different types of behavioural interventions showed results in favour of treatments with some form of contingency management in respect to both reducing drop-outs and lowering cocaine use.

What this review adds to the current knowledge: The systematic review identified as many as 27 trials with a considerable number of participants. The presence of heterogeneity hindered the possibility of pooling the results. However, some types of contingency management techniques are a good treatment approach, provided they can be replicated in a particular therapeutic setting.

Main limitations: Differences in psychiatric and substance use diagnosis, study quality and design, quality of reporting, definitions of outcome variables, varying amounts of subjects in study and varying amounts of psychotherapy provided (ranging from two sessions to 9 months of treatment) produced a considerable amount of heterogeneity.

The future: Randomised trials with adequate sample size and follow-up are needed to further explore the current available evidence for psychosocial interventions for treating psychostimulant dependence. Some promising interventions depicted in this review need further exploration and applicability to other settings and treatment programmes. In addition, the optimal dose and duration of any psychosocial treatment need further investigation.

Reference

1 Knapp WP, Soares BG, Farrel M, Lima MS. Psychosocial interventions for cocaine and psychostimulant amphetamines related disorders. Cochrane Database Syst Rev. 2007(3):CD003023.

Chapter 27 **Antidepressants for cocaine dependence**[1]

Review question: Are antidepressants effective for cocaine dependence and cocaine abuse?

What is known of this topic: Cocaine use is a disorder that can lead to dependence and generate medical and social problems. No pharmacological treatment of proven efficacy exists for cocaine dependence. According to pre-clinical findings and theoretical foundations, antidepressant pharmacotherapy, by augmenting monoamine levels, may alleviate cocaine abstinence symptomatology, as well as relieve dysphoria and associated craving by general antidepressant action.

Summary answer: Evidence data do not support the efficacy of antidepressants in the treatment of cocaine abuse and dependence.

Last assessment date: 9 November 2011

Objectives: To investigate the efficacy and acceptability of antidepressants alone or in combination with any psychosocial intervention for the treatment of cocaine dependence and problematic cocaine use. *Primary outcomes*: Drop-outs, number and type of side effects experienced during the treatment, use of primary substance and results at follow-up. *Other outcomes*: Compliance, craving and severity of dependence as measured by validated scales, amount of cocaine use, psychiatric symptoms and psychological distress diagnosed using standard criteria, quality of life measures and death.

Study population: Cocaine-dependent patients. People younger than 18 years and pregnant women were excluded due to the substantially different approach to clinical management of these people.

Alcohol and Drug Misuse: A Cochrane Handbook, First Edition. Iosief Abraha and Cristina Cusi.
© 2012 John Wiley & Sons, Ltd. Published 2012 by John Wiley & Sons, Ltd.

Search strategy: The Cochrane Library, PubMed, EMBASE, CINAHL (July 2011) and researchers for unpublished trials.

Results: Thirty-seven studies with 3551 participants were included.

- *Antidepressants versus placebo*: Results for drop-outs did not show evidence of difference (31 studies, 2819 participants, RR 1.03 (CI 95% 0.93–1.14)). There was a trend in favour of antidepressants in the 3-week abstinence rate (eight studies, 942 participants, RR 1.22 (CI 95% 0.99–1.51)). Considering studies involving only tricyclics (five studies with 367 participants) or only desipramine (four studies with 254 participants), the evidence was in favour of antidepressants. However, when selecting only studies with operationally defined diagnostic criteria, statistical significance favouring antidepressants, as well as the trend for significance shown by the full sample, disappeared. Looking at safety issues, the results did not show evidence of differences (the number of patients withdrawn for medical reasons, 13 studies, 1396 participants, RR 1.39 (CI 95% 0.91–2.12)). Subgroup analysis considering length of the trial, associated opioid dependence or associated psychosocial interventions as confounding factors failed to show consistent and statistically significant differences in favour of antidepressants.
- *Antidepressants versus other drugs*: Comparing antidepressants with dopamine agonists or with anticonvulsants, no evidence of differences was shown on drop-outs and on other outcomes (abstinence from cocaine use or adverse events).

What this review adds to the current knowledge: Partially positive results obtained on secondary outcome measures, such as depression severity, do not seem to be associated with an effect on direct indicators of cocaine dependence. Despite the abundant number of published studies, antidepressants cannot be considered a mainstay of treatment for unselected cocaine dependents.

Main limitations: The overall quality of the studies was low: although 78% were double-blind studies, only 47% were judged with low risk of bias for the sequence generation, 36% for the allocation concealment and 30% did not address incomplete outcome data. Moreover, 25% of studies did not specify how compliance with medication intake was monitored. However, after excluding studies with a high risk of bias, the results did not change substantially.

The future: The review authors suggest that, given the number of published studies, research on desipramine should not be encouraged. The generic belonging to the antidepressant pharmacological classes is not a good reason for testing medications in clinical trials for the treatment of cocaine dependence; and the issue of the efficacy of antidepressants for patients with cocaine dependence and comorbid depressive disorder deserves further investigation.

Reference

1 Pani PP, Trogu E, Vecchi S, Amato L. Antidepressants for cocaine dependence and problematic cocaine use. Cochrane Database of Syst Rev. 2011(12):CD002950. Epub 2011/12/14.

Chapter 28 **Antipsychotic medications for cocaine dependence**[1]

Review question: Are antipsychotic medications effective for cocaine dependence?

What is known of this topic: Cocaine dependence is a major public health problem that is characterised by an array of medical and psychosocial complications. Antipsychotic medications for cocaine dependence can be a potential source of treatment since use of cocaine can induce hallucinations and paranoia that mimic psychosis.

Summary: Evidence is scarce to recommend the use of antipsychotic medications for the treatment of hallucinations and paranoia in cocaine-dependent subjects.

Last assessment date: 9 May 2007

Objectives: To evaluate the efficacy and the acceptability of antipsychotic medications for cocaine dependence. *Primary outcomes*: Drop-outs from the treatment, side effects, use of primary substance and results at follow-up as number of participants using cocaine at follow-up. *Other outcomes*: Compliance, craving, severity of dependence, amount of cocaine use, psychiatric symptoms or psychological distress.

Study population: Cocaine-dependent patients as diagnosed by the *Diagnostic and Statistical Manual of Mental Disorders* (DSM-IV-TR) or by specialists.

Search strategy: MEDLINE, EMBASE, CINAHL, the Cochrane Drug and Alcohol Group's Specialised Register (October 2006), reference lists of trials, electronic sources of on-going trials (National Research Register, metaRegister of Controlled Trials and Clinical Trials.gov) and conference proceedings.

Alcohol and Drug Misuse: A Cochrane Handbook, First Edition. Iosief Abraha and Cristina Cusi.
© 2012 John Wiley & Sons, Ltd. Published 2012 by John Wiley & Sons, Ltd.

Results: Seven studies with 293 participants were included.

No significant differences were found for any of the efficacy measures comparing any antipsychotic with placebo.

Risperidone resulted superior to placebo in reducing the number of drop-outs in four studies with 178 participants, RR 0.77 (95% CI 0.77–0.98).

Most of the included studies did not report helpful data on important outcomes such as side effects, use of cocaine during treatment and craving. Trials on olanzapine and haloperidol were inadequately powered to give conclusive results.

What this review adds to the current knowledge: Seven trials that evaluated antipsychotic medications for cocaine dependence were identified. Most results were not in favour of antipsychotic medications except for risperidone which resulted effectively in reducing the number of drop-outs.

Main limitations: Outcome reporting bias and inadequate sample size.

The future: Larger randomised investigations analysing relevant outcomes and achieving greater consistency in outcomes and better reporting to enable meaningful cumulative analysis in the future are needed.

Review: Antipsychotic medications for cocaine dependence
Comparison: 2 Risperidone versus Placebo
Outcome: 1 Dropouts

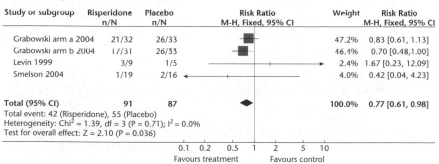

Study or subgroup	Risperidone n/N	Placebo n/N	Risk Ratio M-H, Fixed, 95% CI	Weight	Risk Ratio M-H, Fixed, 95% CI
Grabowski arm a 2004	21/32	26/33		47.2%	0.83 [0.61, 1.13]
Grabowski arm b 2004	17/31	26/33		46.1%	0.70 [0.48,1.00]
Levin 1999	3/9	1/5		2.4%	1.67 [0.23, 12.09]
Smelson 2004	1/19	2/16		4.0%	0.42 [0.04, 4.23]
Total (95% CI)	91	87		100.0%	0.77 [0.61, 0.98]

Total event: 42 (Risperidone), 55 (Placebo)
Heterogeneity: Chi^2 = 1.39, df = 3 (P = 0.71); I^2 = 0.0%
Test for overall effect: Z = 2.10 (P = 0.036)

0.1 0.2 0.5   1   2   5   10
Favours treatment   Favours control

Figure 28.1 Risperidone versus placebo, outcome: drop-outs. Reproduced from Amato L, Minozzi S, Pani PP, Davoli M. Antipsychotic medications for cocaine dependence. Cochrane Database Syst Rev. 2007(3):CD006306, with permission from John Wiley & Sons Ltd. Copyright © 2007 The Cochrane Collaboration.

Reference

1 Amato L, Minozzi S, Pani PP, Davoli M. Antipsychotic medications for cocaine dependence. Cochrane Database Syst Rev. 2007(3):CD006306. Epub 2007/07/20.

Chapter 29 **Anticonvulsants for cocaine dependence**[1]

Review question: What is the efficacy of anticonvulsants for cocaine dependence?

What is known of this topic: Cocaine dependence is a major public health problem that is characterised by a range of medical and psychosocial complications. Anticonvulsants have been considered potential candidates for the treatment of addiction based on the hypothesis that seizure kindling-like mechanisms contribute to addiction.

Summary: Current evidence is limited to support the clinical use of anticonvulsant medications in the treatment of cocaine dependence.

Last assessment date: 6 February 2008

Objectives: To evaluate the efficacy and the acceptability of anticonvulsants for cocaine dependence. *Primary outcomes*: Drop-outs from the treatment, acceptability of the treatment, use of primary substance and results at follow-up as number of participants using cocaine at follow-up. *Other outcomes*: Compliance, craving, severity of dependence as amount of cocaine use, psychiatric symptoms and psychological distress.

Study population: Cocaine-dependent patients as diagnosed by the *Diagnostic and Statistical Manual of Mental Disorders* (DSM-IV-TR) or by specialists.

Search strategy: The Cochrane Drugs and Alcohol Group's specialised register (Issue 4, 2007), MEDLINE, EMBASE and CINAHL (March 2007).

Results: Fifteen studies with 1066 participants were included. The anticonvulsants assessed in the included studies were carbamazepine, gabapentin, lamotrigine, phenytoin, tiagabine, topiramate and valproate.

Alcohol and Drug Misuse: A Cochrane Handbook, First Edition. Iosief Abraha and Cristina Cusi.
© 2012 John Wiley & Sons, Ltd. Published 2012 by John Wiley & Sons, Ltd.

- *Any anticonvulsants versus placebo (12 studies with 793 participants)*: There was no statistical difference, RR 1.05 (95% CI 0.92–1.19).
- *Single anticonvulsants versus placebo*: In two studies (81 participants), gabapentin resulted inferior to placebo in diminishing the number of drop-outs, RR 3.56 (95% CI 1.07–11.82).

In two other studies (56 participants), phenythoin resulted inferior to placebo for side effects, RR 2.12 (95% CI 1.08–4.17).

The remaining single comparisons reported results that were not statistically significant.

What this review adds to the current knowledge: Caution is needed when assessing results from a limited number of small clinical trials. At present there is no evidence supporting the clinical use of anticonvulsant medications in the treatment of cocaine dependence.

Main limitations: Inconsistency in the results across the studies and limited sample size. Several studies were at high risk of bias due to potential selection bias and detection bias.

The future: To obtain randomised trials of high quality and to enable meaningful cumulative analysis, researchers should achieve greater consistency in outcomes measure (drop-out and use of cocaine measured as number of subjects abstinent at the end of treatment).

Reference

1 Minozzi S, Amato L, Davoli M, Farrell M, Lima Reisser ΛΛ, Pani PP, *et al.* Anticonvulsants for cocaine dependence. Cochrane Database Syst Rev. 2008(2):CD006754. Epub 2008/04/22.

Chapter 30 **Dopamine agonists for cocaine dependence**[1]

Review question: Can dopamine agonists be effective for the treatment of cocaine dependence?

What is known of this topic: Cocaine use is a disorder that can lead to dependence and generate medical and social problems. No pharmacological treatment of proven efficacy exists for cocaine dependence. Manipulation of dopamine transmission in the reward circuitry of the brain has been seen as the mainstay of the development of new medications for the treatment of cocaine dependence. Specifically, dopamine agonists acting on brain dopamine transporters or brain dopamine receptors may alleviate cocaine abstinence symptoms and reduce craving and the risk of relapse.

Summary answer: Current evidence from randomised trials does not support the use of dopamine agonists for treating cocaine dependence.

Last assessment date: 12 October 2011

Objectives: To investigate the efficacy and acceptability of dopamine agonists alone or in combination with any psychosocial intervention for the treatment of cocaine use and dependence. *Primary outcomes*: Completion of treatment, acceptability of the treatment as number of participants experiencing adverse effects, drop-outs due to adverse effects, abstinence self-reported and/or number of participants with urine samples negative for cocaine and results at follow-up as number of participants abstinent at follow-up. *Other outcomes*: Craving, severity of dependence, clinical global valuation and psychiatric or psychological symptoms.

Study population: Cocaine users or dependents as diagnosed by the *Diagnostic and Statistical Manual of Mental Disorders* (DSM-III-R, DSM-IV and DSM-IV-TR) or by specialists. Participants younger than 18 years and preg-

Alcohol and Drug Misuse: A Cochrane Handbook, First Edition. Iosief Abraha and Cristina Cusi.
© 2012 John Wiley & Sons, Ltd. Published 2012 by John Wiley & Sons, Ltd.

nant women were excluded. People with comorbid mental health conditions were included and considered in subgroup analysis.

Search strategy: The Cochrane Drugs and Alcohol Group Specialized Register, PubMed, EMBASE, CINAHL, PsycINFO (June 2011); contacted researchers for unpublished trials

Results: Twenty-three studies with 2066 participants were included.

- *Any dopamine agonist versus placebo*: Placebo performed better for severity of dependence (four studies with 232 participants, SMD 0.43 (95% CI 0.15 to 0.71)), depression (five studies with 322 participants, SMD 0.42 (95% CI 0.19 to 0.65)) and abstinence at follow-up, RR 0.57 (95% CI 0.35–0.93). No statistically significant difference for the other outcomes was considered.

Comparing amantadine versus placebo, results never gain statistical significance, but there was a trend in favour of amantadine for drop-outs and depression. Results on adverse events and depression were in favour of placebo, although the differences did not reach statistical significance.

Comparing bromocriptine and Ldopa/Carbidopa versus placebo, results never reached statistical significance.

Comparing amantadine versus antidepressants, antidepressants performed better for abstinence. The other two outcomes considered did not show statistically significant differences, although drop-outs and adverse events tended to be more common in the antidepressant group.

What this review adds to the current knowledge: A considerable number of trials were retrieved from the medical literature. Despite the theoretical foundations on which the use of dopamine agonists for the treatment of cocaine dependence is based on, current evidence from randomised trials does not support the use of dopamine agonists for treating cocaine dependence. Even the potential benefit of combining a dopamine agonist with a more potent psychosocial intervention, which was suggested by the previous *Cochrane Review*,[2] is not supported by the results of this updated review.

Main limitations: The quality of evidence, assessed according to the GRADE method, may be judged as moderate for the efficacy of any dopamine agonist versus placebo and as moderate to high for amantadine versus placebo and versus antidepressants.

The future: It is unlikely that future studies can change the conclusions of the review.

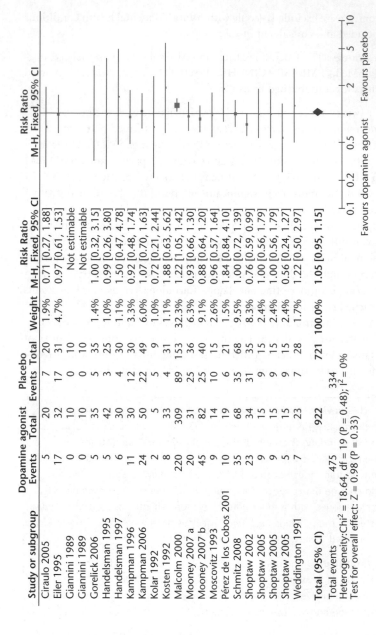

Study or subgroup	Dopamine agonist Events	Dopamine agonist Total	Placebo Events	Placebo Total	Weight	Risk Ratio M-H, Fixed, 95% CI
Ciraulo 2005	5	20	7	20	1.9%	0.71 [0.27, 1.88]
Eiler 1995	17	32	17	31	4.7%	0.97 [0.61, 1.53]
Giannini 1989	0	10	0	10		Not estimable
Giannini 1989	0	10	0	10		Not estimable
Gorelick 2006	5	35	5	35	1.4%	1.00 [0.32, 3.15]
Handelsman 1995	5	42	3	25	1.0%	0.99 [0.26, 3.80]
Handelsman 1997	6	30	4	30	1.1%	1.50 [0.47, 4.78]
Kampman 1996	11	30	12	30	3.3%	0.92 [0.48, 1.74]
Kampman 2006	24	50	22	49	6.0%	1.07 [0.70, 1.63]
Kolar 1992	2	5	5	9	1.0%	0.72 [0.21, 2.44]
Kosten 1992	8	33	4	31	1.1%	1.88 [0.63, 5.62]
Malcolm 2000	220	309	89	153	32.3%	1.22 [1.05, 1.42]
Mooney 2007 a	20	31	25	36	6.3%	0.93 [0.66, 1.30]
Mooney 2007 b	45	82	25	40	9.1%	0.88 [0.64, 1.20]
Moscovitz 1993	9	14	10	15	2.6%	0.96 [0.57, 1.64]
Pérez de los Cobos 2001	10	19	6	21	1.5%	1.84 [0.84, 4.10]
Schmitz 2008	35	68	35	68	9.5%	1.00 [0.72, 1.39]
Shoptaw 2002	23	34	31	35	8.3%	0.76 [0.59, 0.99]
Shoptaw 2005	9	15	9	15	2.4%	1.00 [0.56, 1.79]
Shoptaw 2005	9	15	9	15	2.4%	1.00 [0.56, 1.79]
Shoptaw 2005	5	15	9	15	2.4%	0.56 [0.24, 1.27]
Weddington 1991	7	23	7	28	1.7%	1.22 [0.50, 2.97]
Total (95% CI)		**922**		**721**	**100.0%**	**1.05 [0.95, 1.15]**

Total events 475 334
Heterogeneity:Chi^2 = 18.64, df = 19 (P = 0.48); I^2 = 0%
Test for overall effect: Z = 0.98 (P = 0.33)

0.1 0.2 0.5 1 2 5 10
Favours dopamine agonist   Favours placebo

Figure 30.1 Dopamine agonists versus placebo for the treatment of cocaine dependence: Dropouts. Reproduced from Soares BG, Lima MS, Reisser AA, Farrell M. Dopamine agonists for cocaine dependence. Cochrane Database Syst Rev. 2003(2):CD003352, with permission from John Wiley & Sons Ltd. Copyright © 2003 The Cochrane Collaboration.

References

1 Castells X, Casas M, Perez-Mana C, Roncero C, Vidal X, Capella D. Efficacy of psychostimulant drugs for cocaine dependence. Cochrane Database Syst Rev. 2010(2):CD007380. Epub 2010/02/19.
2 Soares BG, Lima MS, Reisser AA, Farrell M. Dopamine agonists for cocaine dependence. Cochrane Database Syst Rev. 2003(2):CD003352. Epub 2003/06/14.

Chapter 31 **Disulfiram for the treatment of cocaine dependence**[1]

Review question: Is disulfiram effective for the treatment of cocaine dependence?

What is known of this topic: Cocaine use is a disorder that can lead to dependence and generate medical, psychological and social problems. No pharmacological treatment of proven efficacy exists for cocaine dependence. Disulfiram is a compound that has the ability to interfere with enzymes involved in the metabolism of cerebral monoamines. In particular by inhibiting the dopamine beta-hydroxylase, it may favourably influence the functioning of the mesolimbic circuits disrupted by cocaine addiction.

Summary: The evidence is low to recommend disulfiram for the treatment of cocaine dependence.

Last assessment date: 13 October 2009

Objectives: To evaluate the efficacy and the safety of disulfiram for cocaine dependence. *Primary outcomes*: Drop-outs from the treatment, rates of side effects, use of primary substance and results at follow-up. *Other outcomes*: Compliance, craving, severity of dependence, amount of cocaine use, psychiatric symptoms and psychological distress.

Study population: Cocaine dependents as diagnosed by the *Diagnostic and Statistical Manual of Mental Disorders* (DSM-IV-TR) or by specialists. Participants younger than 18 years and pregnant women were excluded.

Search strategy: PubMed, EMBASE, CINAHL (January 2008), the Cochrane Central Register of Controlled Trials (Issue 1, 2009), reference lists of trials, main electronic sources of on-going trials and conference proceedings.

Alcohol and Drug Misuse: A Cochrane Handbook, First Edition. Iosief Abraha and Cristina Cusi.
© 2012 John Wiley & Sons, Ltd. Published 2012 by John Wiley & Sons, Ltd.

Results: Seven studies with 492 participants were included.

- *Disulfiram versus placebo:* No statistically significant results for drop-outs (RR 0.64, 95% CI 0.35–1.20) even after excluding a trial that had an exaggerated treatment effect in favour of disulfiram (RR 0.34, 95% CI 0.20–0.58) and was responsible for significant heterogeneity. For cocaine use, it was not possible to pool together primary studies. However, only one study (with 20 participants) out of four resulted in favour of disulfiram for the outcome number of weeks abstinence (WMD 4.50, 95% CI 2.93 to 6.07).

- *Disulfiram versus naltrexone:* No statistically significant results for drop-outs but a trend favouring disulfiram from three studies with 131 participants (RR 0.67, 95% CI 0.45–1.01). No significant difference for cocaine use was seen in the only study that considered this outcome.

- *Disulfiram versus no pharmacological treatment:* For cocaine use, only one study with 90 participants reported data that resulted in a statistically significant difference in favour of disulfiram (maximum weeks of consecutive abstinence (WMD 2.10 , 95% CI 0.69 to 3.51) and number of subjects achieving 3 or more weeks of consecutive abstinence (RR 1.88, 95% CI 1.09–3.23)).

What this review adds to the current knowledge: Trials published on disulfiram to assess the effects of disulfiram for cocaine dependence are few. Evidence supporting the clinical use of disulfiram in the treatment of cocaine dependence is low.

Main limitations: Study design of limited quality and small sample size, and the presence of heterogeneity. Outcome reporting bias.

The future: High-quality randomised trials investigating relevant outcomes are needed.

Reference

1 Pani PP, Trogu E, Vacca R, Amato L, Vecchi S, Davoli M. Disulfiram for the treatment of cocaine dependence. Cochrane Database Syst Rev. 2010(1):CD007024. Epub 2010/01/22.

Chapter 32 **Efficacy of psychostimulant drugs for cocaine dependence**[1]

Review question: Are psychostimulants effective for cocaine dependence on cocaine use, sustained cocaine abstinence and retention in treatment?

What is known of this topic: Cocaine use is a disorder that can lead to dependence and generate medical, psychological and social problems. No pharmacological treatment of proven efficacy exists for cocaine dependence. Psychostimulants can be a valid alternative for cocaine dependence.

Summary: At present there is no evidence to recommend psychostimulants for the treatment of cocaine dependence.

Last assessment date: 24 July 2008

Objectives: To assess the efficacy of psychostimulants for cocaine dependence on cocaine use, sustained cocaine abstinence and retention in treatment. *Other outcomes*: The influence of type of drug, comorbid disorders and clinical trial reporting quality over psychostimulant efficacy has also been studied.

Study population: Adult participants meeting criteria for cocaine use or cocaine dependence using *Diagnostic and Statistical Manual of Mental Disorders* (DSM-IV-TR) criteria.

Search strategy: Cochrane Central Register of Controlled Trials, *The Cochrane Library* (Issue 4, 2008), MEDLINE, EMBASE, PsycINFO (January 2009), www.controlled-trials.com, clinicalstudyresults.org and centerwatch.com.

Results: Sixteen studies with 1345 participants were included. Bupropion, dexamphetamine, methylphenidate, modafinil, mazindol, methamphetamine and selegiline were the medications investigated.
- *Any psychostimulant versus placebo*: For the outcome cocaine use, seven studies with 469 participants, there was no statistical difference between the two groups (SMD 0.11, 95% CI −0.07 to 0.29).

Alcohol and Drug Misuse: A Cochrane Handbook, First Edition. Iosief Abraha and Cristina Cusi.
© 2012 John Wiley & Sons, Ltd. Published 2012 by John Wiley & Sons, Ltd.

For the outcome sustained cocaine abstinence, eight studies with 811 participants, there was no statistical difference (RR 0.71, 95% CI 0.50–1.02) though there was a trend in favour to psychostimulants (P = 0.07) with moderate heterogeneity ($I^2 = 32\%$).

For the outcome retention in treatment, there was no significant difference (RR 1.03, 95% CI 0.95–1.12).

No statistical difference was found for the remaining outcomes.

What this review adds to the current knowledge: Sixteen studies investigating the efficacy of psychostimulants for the treatment of cocaine dependence were published. Not all studies evaluated all outcomes except for retention in treatment. Results were not significant to recommend the use of psychostimulants for the treatment of cocaine dependence. However, psychostimulants as an add-on treatment may be beneficial in dual heroin–cocaine dependents who are maintained with methadone.

Main limitations: Attrition and outcome reporting bias.

The future: Although the results were not statistically significant in favour of psychostimulants, these medications may require an intense research activity in the future. Given the high attrition that features cocaine dependence studies, which hampers the validity of any clinical trial, future studies should address incomplete outcome data.

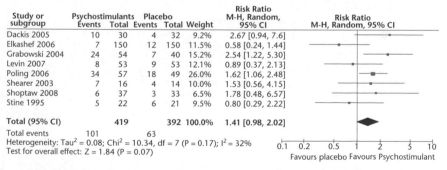

Study or subgroup	Psychostimulants Events	Total	Placebo Events	Total	Weight	Risk Ratio M-H, Random, 95% CI	Risk Ratio M-H, Random, 95% CI
Dackis 2005	10	30	4	32	9.2%	2.67 [0.94, 7.6]	
Elkashef 2006	7	150	12	150	11.5%	0.58 [0.24, 1.44]	
Grabowski 2004	24	54	7	40	15.2%	2.54 [1.22, 5.30]	
Levin 2007	8	53	9	53	12.1%	0.89 [0.37, 2.13]	
Poling 2006	34	57	18	49	26.0%	1.62 [1.06, 2.48]	
Shearer 2003	7	16	4	14	10.0%	1.53 [0.56, 4.15]	
Shoptaw 2008	6	37	3	33	6.5%	1.78 [0.48, 6.57]	
Stine 1995	5	22	6	21	9.5%	0.80 [0.29, 2.22]	
Total (95% CI)		**419**		**392**	**100.0%**	**1.41 [0.98, 2.02]**	
Total events	101		63				

Heterogeneity: Tau^2 = 0.08; Chi^2 = 10.34, df = 7 (P = 0.17); I^2 = 32%
Test for overall effect: Z = 1.84 (P = 0.07)

Favours placebo Favours Psychostimulant

Figure 32.1 Psychostimulants versus placebo, outcome: sustained cocaine abstinence. Reproduced from Castells X, Casas M, Perez-Mana C, Roncero C, Vidal X, Capella D. Efficacy of psychostimulant drugs for cocaine dependence. Cochrane Database Syst Rev. 2010(2):CD007380, with permission from John Wiley & Sons Ltd. Copyright © 2010 The Cochrane Collaboration.

Reference

1 Castells X, Casas M, Perez-Mana C, Roncero C, Vidal X, Capella D. Efficacy of psychostimulant drugs for cocaine dependence. Cochrane Database Syst Rev. 2010(2):CD007380. Epub 2010/02/19.

Chapter 33 **Auricular acupuncture for cocaine dependence**[1]

Review question: Is auricular acupuncture effective for cocaine dependence?

What is known of this topic: Currently, there is no effective treatment available for cocaine dependence. Auricular acupuncture (insertion of acupuncture into a number, usually five, of specific points in the ear) is a widely used treatment for cocaine dependence. A systematic review is needed to address this issue.

Summary: There is currently no evidence that auricular acupuncture is effective for the treatment of cocaine dependence.

Last assessment date: 27 October 2005

Objectives: To determine whether auricular acupuncture is an effective treatment for cocaine dependence, and to investigate whether its effectiveness is influenced by the treatment regimen. *Outcome studied*: Cocaine use, severity of dependence, side effects, attrition from treatment programmes and cocaine craving.

Study population: Participants with cocaine or crack cocaine dependence.

Search strategy: Cochrane Central Register of Controlled Trials, *The Cochrane Library* (Issue 3, 2004), MEDLINE (January 1966 to October 2004), EMBASE (January 1988 to October 2004), PsycINFO (1985 to October 2004), CINAHL (1982 to October 2004), SIGLE (1980 to October 2004) and reference lists of articles.

Results: Seven studies with 1433 participants were included.
- *Auricular acupuncture versus sham acupuncture*: There was no statistical difference in terms of cocaine use in the short term (three studies; RR 1.01,

Alcohol and Drug Misuse: A Cochrane Handbook, First Edition. Iosief Abraha and Cristina Cusi.
© 2012 John Wiley & Sons, Ltd. Published 2012 by John Wiley & Sons, Ltd.

95% CI 0.94–1.08) and in the long term (one study; RR 0.98, 95% CI 0.89–1.09).

• *Auricular acupuncture versus no acupuncture*: There was no statistical difference in the short term (RR 0.99, 95% 0.92 to 1.05; heterogeneity $I^2 = 67.9\%$).

There was no difference also for the outcome cocaine use as self-reported.

No differences between acupuncture and sham acupuncture were found for attrition (RR 1.05, 95% CI 0.89–1.23), or between acupuncture and no acupuncture (RR 1.06, 95% CI 0.90–1.26), neither for any measure of cocaine or other drug use.

Side effects of treatment were not reported by any study.

What this review adds to the current knowledge: Results from this review do not provide sufficient evidence to support the use of acupuncture for the treatment of cocaine dependence.

Main limitations: All studies were of generally low methodological quality that together with the presence of outcome reporting bias may threaten the validity of the conclusions of the present review.

The future: Further research may change the results of the current review. Randomised trials of high methodological quality, adequate sample size and long-term follow-up are warranted.

Reference

1 Gates S, Smith LA, Foxcroft DR. Auricular acupuncture for cocaine dependence. Cochrane Database Syst Rev. 2006(1):CD005192.

Chapter 34 **Psychosocial treatment for opiate dependence**[1]

Review question: Are psychosocial interventions alone effective and acceptable for treating opiate use disorders?

What is known of this topic: Substance use is a social and public health problem; therefore it is a priority to develop effective treatments. Previous Cochrane Reviews have explored the efficacy of pharmacotherapy for opiate dependence. This current review focuses on the role of psychosocial interventions alone for the treatment of opiate dependence. There is some evidence for the effectiveness of psychosocial interventions, but no systematic review has ever been carried out.

Summary: The evidence suggests that psychosocial interventions alone cannot be recommended for opiate-related disorders.

Last assessment date: 8 August 2004

Objectives: To assess the efficacy and acceptability of psychosocial interventions for treating opioid dependence compared to non-psychosocial interventions (pharmacological, placebo or no intervention). *Primary outcome*: Use of primary substance craving, retention in treatment, compliance, relapse at follow-up, mortality, physical health and quality of life.

Study population: People with any clinical diagnosis for opioid dependence, irrespective of pattern, gender, age or nationality. Trials including patients with additional diagnoses such as alcoholism or psychostimulant dependence were also eligible.

Search strategy: The Cochrane Drugs and Alcohol Group's Register of Trials (21 January 2004), the Cochrane Library (2004), MEDLINE, LILACS, EMBASE, PsycINFO (2003), reference searching, personal communication, conference abstracts, unpublished trials and book chapters on treatment of opioid dependence.

Alcohol and Drug Misuse: A Cochrane Handbook, First Edition. Iosief Abraha and Cristina Cusi.
© 2012 John Wiley & Sons, Ltd. Published 2012 by John Wiley & Sons, Ltd.

Results: Five trials involving 389 participants were included.

These studies analysed Contingency Management, Brief Reinforcement Based Intensive Outpatient Therapy coupled with Contingency Management, Cue Exposure therapy, Alternative Programme for Methadone Maintenance Treatment Programme Drop-outs (MMTP) and Enhanced Outreach-Counselling Programme. All the treatments were studied against the control (standard) treatment; therefore it was not possible to identify which type of psychosocial therapy was most effective.

The main findings were that both Enhanced Outreach Counselling and Brief Reinforcement Based Intensive Outpatient Therapy coupled with Contingency Management had significantly better outcomes than standard therapy regarding relapse to opioid use, re-enrolment in treatment and retention in treatment. At 1-month and 3-month follow-up, the effects of Brief Reinforcement Based Intensive Outpatient Therapy were not sustained. There was no further follow-up of the Enhanced Outreach-Counselling Programme. The Alternative Programme for MMTP Drop-outs and the behavioural therapies of Cue Exposure and Contingency Management alone were no better than the control. As the studies were heterogeneous, it was not possible to pool the results and perform a meta-analysis.

What this review adds to the current knowledge: The available data are on a very small scale, and at present psychosocial treatments alone are not adequately proved treatment modalities or superior to any other type of treatment.

Main limitations: Trials were of limited sample size and presented limited methodological quality. In addition, the definitions of the outcome studied were highly heterogeneous, which limited the performance of meta-analysis.

The future: Large randomised trials with sound methodology and longer follow-ups to examine whether psychosocial interventions alone help patients with opioid use disorders are needed. These studies would need to take account of the study setting as this may have a confounding effect on the results. In addition, they need to investigate whether one psychosocial intervention is more effective than another and whether the effectiveness depends upon personality factors, psychiatric comorbid diagnosis, length of therapy time, severity of illicit drug use or any other factors.

Reference

1 Mayet S, Farrell M, Ferri M, Amato L, Davoli M. Psychosocial treatment for opiate abuse and dependence. Cochrane Database Syst Rev. 2005(1):CD004330.

Chapter 35 **Psychosocial and pharmacological treatments versus pharmacological treatments for opioid detoxification**[1]

Review question: Are psychosocial associated with pharmacological interventions effective in helping patients to complete the treatment, reduce the use of substances and improve health and social status?

What is known of this topic: Several pharmacological approaches are available for opioid detoxification. However, the majority of subjects relapse to heroin use, and relapses are a substantial problem in the rehabilitation of heroin users. Some studies have suggested that the sorts of symptoms which are most distressing to addicts during detoxification are psychological rather than physiological symptoms associated with withdrawal.

Summary: Psychosocial treatments offered in addition to pharmacological detoxification treatments are effective in terms of completion of treatment, use of opiate, results at follow-up and compliance.

Last assessment date: 17 July 2011

Objectives: To evaluate the effectiveness of any psychosocial plus any pharmacological interventions versus any pharmacological intervention alone for opioid detoxification, in helping patients to complete the treatment, reduce the use of substances and improve health and social status. *Other outcomes*: Compliance as clinical absences during the study period, use of other drugs, mortality and engagement in further treatment.

Study population: Opiate addicts undergoing any psychosocial intervention associated with any pharmacological intervention aimed at opioid detoxification. People younger than 18 years and pregnant women were excluded.

Alcohol and Drug Misuse: A Cochrane Handbook, First Edition. Iosief Abraha and Cristina Cusi.
© 2012 John Wiley & Sons, Ltd. Published 2012 by John Wiley & Sons, Ltd.

Search strategy: The Cochrane Drugs and Alcohol Group's trials register (June 2011), *The Cochrane Library* (Issue 6, 2011), PUBMED, EMBASE, CINAHL (June 2008), PsycINFO (April 2003) and reference lists of articles.

Results: Eleven studies with 1592 participants were included.

The studies considered five different psychosocial interventions and two pharmacological treatments (methadone and buprenorphine). Compared to any pharmacological treatment alone, the association of any psychosocial with any pharmacological intervention was shown to significantly reduce drop-outs (RR 0.71, 95% CI 0.59–0.85), use of opiate during the treatment (RR 0.82, 95% CI 0.71–0.93) and at follow-up (RR 0.66, 95% IC 0.53–0.82) and clinical absences during the treatment (RR 0.48, 95% CI 0.38–0.59). Moreover, with the evidence currently available, there are no data supporting a single psychosocial approach.

What this review adds to the current knowledge: Psychosocial treatment added to pharmacological detoxification treatment is effective in terms of completion of treatment, use of opiate, results at follow-up and compliance.

Main limitations: Most of the studies had unclear allocation concealment or did not report information on loss to follow-up. In addition, there was heterogeneity of the assessment of outcomes.

The future: Further studies are unlikely to change the current recommendation. However, highly standardised definitions of the outcomes measured are needed.

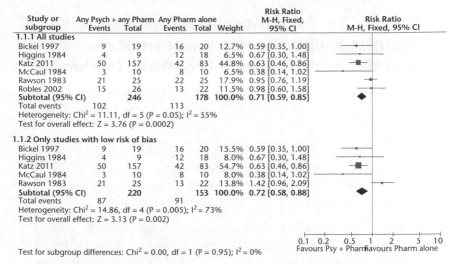

Study or subgroup	Any Psych + any Pharm		Any Pharm alone			Risk Ratio M-H, Fixed, 95% CI	Risk Ratio M-H, Fixed, 95% CI
	Events	Total	Events	Total	Weight		
1.1.1 All studies							
Bickel 1997	9	19	16	20	12.7%	0.59 [0.35, 1.00]	
Higgins 1984	4	9	12	18	6.5%	0.67 [0.30, 1.48]	
Katz 2011	50	157	42	83	44.8%	0.63 [0.46, 0.86]	
McCaul 1984	3	10	8	10	6.5%	0.38 [0.14, 1.02]	
Rawson 1983	21	25	22	25	17.9%	0.95 [0.76, 1.19]	
Robles 2002	15	26	13	22	11.5%	0.98 [0.60, 1.58]	
Subtotal (95% CI)		246		178	100.0%	0.71 [0.59, 0.85]	
Total events	102		113				
Heterogeneity: Chi^2 = 11.11, df = 5 (P = 0.05); I^2 = 55%							
Test for overall effect: Z = 3.76 (P = 0.0002)							
1.1.2 Only studies with low risk of bias							
Bickel 1997	9	19	16	20	15.5%	0.59 [0.35, 1.00]	
Higgins 1984	4	9	12	18	8.0%	0.67 [0.30, 1.48]	
Katz 2011	50	157	42	83	54.7%	0.63 [0.46, 0.86]	
McCaul 1984	3	10	8	10	8.0%	0.38 [0.14, 1.02]	
Rawson 1983	21	25	13	22	13.8%	1.42 [0.96, 2.09]	
Subtotal (95% CI)		220		153	100.0%	0.72 [0.58, 0.88]	
Total events	87		91				
Heterogeneity: Chi^2 = 14.86, df = 4 (P = 0.005); I^2 = 73%							
Test for overall effect: Z = 3.13 (P = 0.002)							

Test for subgroup differences: Chi^2 = 0.00, df = 1 (P = 0.95); I^2 = 0%

0.1 0.2 0.5 1 2 5 10
Favours Psy + Pharm Favours Pharm alone

Figure 35.1 Any psychosocial plus any pharmacological treatments versus any pharmacological alone, outcome: drop-outs. Reproduced from Amato L, Minozzi S, Davoli M, Vecchi S, Ferri MM, Mayet S. Psychosocial and pharmacological treatments versus pharmacological treatments for opioid detoxification. Cochrane Database Syst Rev. 2008(3):CD005031, with permission from John Wiley & Sons Ltd. Copyright © 2008 The Cochrane Collaboration.

Reference

1 Amato L, Minozzi S, Davoli M, Vecchi S, Ferri MM, Mayet S. Psychosocial and pharmacological treatments versus pharmacological treatments for opioid detoxification. Cochrane Database Syst Rev. 2008(3):CD005031.

Chapter 36 **Psychosocial combined with agonist maintenance treatments versus agonist maintenance treatments alone for treatment of opioid dependence**[1]

Review question: Are psychosocial support added to a maintenance treatment effective for opiate dependence (in terms of retention in treatment, use of substances, health and social status) with respect to standard agonist treatment?

What is known of this topic: Several pharmacological approaches are available for opioid detoxification. However, the majority of subjects relapse to heroin use, and relapses are a substantial problem in the rehabilitation of heroin users. Questions remain, however, about the efficacy of additional psychosocial services offered by most maintenance programmes.

Summary: Adding any psychosocial support to maintenance treatments improves the number of participants abstinent at follow-up; however, there were no significant differences for the remaining outcomes.

Last assessment date: 31 July 2011

Objectives: To evaluate the effectiveness of any psychosocial plus any agonist maintenance treatment versus standard agonist treatment for opiate dependence. *Primary outcomes*: Retention in treatment, abstinence by primary substance measured as number of participants with consecutive negative urinalysis for at least 3 weeks and results at follow-up measured as number of participants who are still in treatment at the end of follow-up or opioid abstinent at the end of follow-up. *Other outcomes*: Compliance, craving, psychiatric symptoms, psychological distress, quality of life, severity of dependence and death.

Alcohol and Drug Misuse: A Cochrane Handbook, First Edition. Iosief Abraha and Cristina Cusi.
© 2012 John Wiley & Sons, Ltd. Published 2012 by John Wiley & Sons, Ltd.

Study population: Opiate addicts undergoing any psychosocial support associated with any agonist maintenance intervention.

Search strategy: The Cochrane Drugs and Alcohol Group's trials register (June 2011), *The Cochrane Library* (Issue 6, 2011), PUBMED, EMBASE, CINAHL (2011), PsycINFO (2003) and reference list of articles.

Results: Thirty-five studies with 4319 participants were included.

Thirteen different psychosocial interventions were considered. Comparing any psychosocial plus any maintenance pharmacological treatment to standard maintenance treatment, results do not show benefit for retention in treatment (27 studies with 3124 participants; RR 1.03, 95% CI 0.98–1.07), abstinence by opiate during the treatment (eight studies with 1002 participants; RR 1.12, 95% CI 0.92–11.37), compliance (three studies; WMD 0.43, 95% CI −0.05 to 0.92), psychiatric symptoms (three studies; WMD 0.02, −0.28 to 0.31), depression (three studies; WMD −1.70, 95% CI −3.91 to 0.51) and results at the end of follow-up as number of participants still in treatment (three studies with 250 participants; RR 0.90, 95% CI 0.77–1.07) and participants abstinent for opioid use (three studies with 181 participants; RR 1.15, 95% CI 0.98–1.36). Comparing the different psychosocial approaches, results are never statistically significant for all the comparisons and outcomes.

What this review adds to the current knowledge: The present evidence suggests that adding psychosocial support does not change the effectiveness of retention in treatment. Nor does it result in a clear reduction in opiate use during treatment. However, the number of participants abstinent at the end of follow-up and continuous weeks of abstinence showed a benefit in favour of the associated treatment.

Main limitations: Studies were of limited sample size.

The future: This review showed that psychosocial interventions can be evaluated in the context of randomised controlled trials. Future trials with adequate sample size and sound methodology could be considered with clearly defined experimental interventions and outcomes.

Reference

1 Amato L, Minozzi S, Davoli M, Vecchi S, Ferri MM, Mayet S. Psychosocial combined with agonist maintenance treatments versus agonist maintenance treatments alone for treatment of opioid dependence. Cochrane Database Syst Rev. 2008 (4):CD004147.

Chapter 37 Alpha$_2$-adrenergic agonists for the management of opioid withdrawal[1]

Review question: Are alpha$_2$-adrenergic agonists effective in the management of opioid withdrawal?

What is known of this topic: Dependence on opioid drugs (heroin and methadone) is a major health and social issue in many societies. Withdrawal is the first step for many forms of longer term treatment in opioid-dependent subjects. The treatment involves the use of medication to reduce withdrawal symptoms associated with gradual or abrupt cessation of opioid medication. Relapse to opioid use following detoxification remains high and rates of completion of withdrawal tend to be low, making follow-up treatment important. The alpha$_2$-adrenergic agonists (e.g. clonidine and lofexidine) act centrally to moderate the symptoms of noradrenergic hyperactivity. Thus these drugs can be a non-opioid alternative for managing withdrawal since they can ameliorate some signs and symptoms of withdrawal.

Summary: Clonidine and lofexidine are more effective than placebo for the management of withdrawal from heroin or methadone. Lofexidine has less effect on blood pressure but otherwise has similar efficacy to clonidine. The severity of withdrawal managed with clonidine or lofexidine is similar to withdrawal managed with reducing doses of methadone, but withdrawal signs and symptoms occur earlier. Clonidine is associated with more adverse effects than reducing doses of methadone.

Last assessment date: 26 October 2008

Objectives: To assess the effectiveness of alpha$_2$-adrenergic agonists compared to reducing doses of methadone or symptomatic medications, or with comparison of different alpha$_2$-adrenergic agonists, for the management of the acute phase of opioid withdrawal. *Other outcomes*: Intensity of signs and

Alcohol and Drug Misuse: A Cochrane Handbook, First Edition. Iosief Abraha and Cristina Cusi.
© 2012 John Wiley & Sons, Ltd. Published 2012 by John Wiley & Sons, Ltd.

symptoms and overall withdrawal experienced, duration of treatment, occurrence of adverse effects and completion of treatment.

Study population: Primarily opioid-dependent participants who underwent managed withdrawal.

Search strategy: Cochrane Central Register of Controlled Trials (Issue 3, 2008), MEDLINE (July 2008), EMBASE, PsycINFO (August 2008) and reference lists of articles.

Results: Twenty-four studies (21 randomised trials), involving 1631 participants, met the inclusion criteria. Thirteen studies compared a treatment regime based on an alpha$_2$-adrenergic agonist with one based on reducing doses of methadone.

- *Alpha$_2$-adrenergic agonists (clonidine or lofexidine) versus placebo (three trials included)*: Alpha$_2$-adrenergic agonists are more effective than placebo in ameliorating withdrawal, and are associated with significantly higher rates of completion (RR 0.53, 95% CI 0.36–0.78) of treatment despite higher rates of adverse effects.
- *Clonidine or lofexidine versus methadone*: There were no significant differences between alpha$_2$-adrenergic agonists and tapered methadone for the outcomes unacceptably high withdrawals (four studies; RR 1.46, 95% CI 0.86–2.46), duration of treatment (three studies; SMD −1.07, 95% CI −1.31 to −0.83) and retention in treatment (three studies; RR 0.81, 95% CI 0.64–1.04). Alpha$_2$-adrenergic agonists were associated with more adverse effects than reducing doses of methadone (RR 2.13, 95% CI 1.30–3.48). Lofexidine does not reduce blood pressure to the same extent as clonidine, but is otherwise similar to clonidine.

What this review adds to the current knowledge: Despite clonidine and lofexidine being more effective than placebo in ameliorating withdrawal, when compared to methadone alpha$_2$-adrenergic agonist treatment does not seem to give advantage with respect to methadone. While with alpha$_2$-adrenergic agonist treatment, the signs and symptoms of withdrawal occurred earlier, with reducing doses of methadone, the signs and symptoms of withdrawal did not become apparent until methadone doses approached zero.

Main limitations: Diversity in study design, assessment and reporting of outcomes limited the extent of quantitative analysis.

The future: Further studies may change the current knowledge of this issue.

98 Drugs

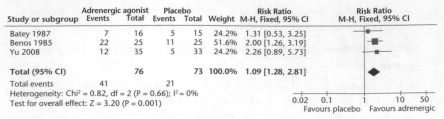

Study or subgroup	Adrenergic agonist Events	Total	Placebo Events	Total	Weight	Risk Ratio M-H, Fixed, 95% CI
Batey 1987	7	16	5	15	24.2%	1.31 [0.53, 3.25]
Benos 1985	22	25	11	25	51.6%	2.00 [1.26, 3.19]
Yu 2008	12	35	5	33	24.2%	2.26 [0.89, 5.73]
Total (95% CI)		76		73	100.0%	1.09 [1.28, 2.81]
Total events	41		21			

Heterogeneity: Chi² = 0.82, df = 2 (P = 0.66); I² = 0%
Test for overall effect: Z = 3.20 (P = 0.001)

Figure 37.1 Adrenergic agonist versus placebo, outcome: treatment completion. Reproduced from Gowing L, Farrell M, Ali R, White JM. Alpha2-adrenergic agonists for the management of opioid withdrawal. Cochrane Database Syst Rev. 2009(2):CD002024, with permission from John Wiley & Sons Ltd. Copyright © 2009 The Cochrane Collaboration.

Reference

1 Gowing L, Farrell M, Ali R, White JM. Alpha$_2$-adrenergic agonists for the management of opioid withdrawal. Cochrane Database Syst Rev. 2009(2):CD002024. Epub 2009/04/17.

Chapter 38 **Buprenorphine for the management of opioid withdrawal**[1]

Review question: Is buprenorphine effective in the management of opioid withdrawal?

What is known of this topic: Managed withdrawal from opioid dependence is an essential first step for drug-free treatment. The treatment requires suppression of withdrawal with methadone and gradual reduction of the methadone dose. However, relapse to opioid use following detoxification remains high and rates of completion of withdrawal tend to be low. The relative efficacy of an alpha$_2$-adrenergic agonist, clonidine, to ameliorate some signs and symptoms of withdrawal led to widespread use of this drug as a non-opioid alternative for managing withdrawal. However, the use of clonidine was limited by adverse effects of sedation and hypotension. Such limitation led to a sustained exploration of a variety of alternative approaches, including buprenorphine.

Summary: Buprenorphine is more effective than clonidine or lofexidine for the management of opioid withdrawal. Buprenorphine may offer some advantages over methadone, at least in inpatient settings, in terms of quicker resolution of withdrawal symptoms and possibly slightly higher rates of completion of withdrawal.

Last assessment date: 17 November 2008

Objectives: To assess the effectiveness of buprenorphine to manage opioid withdrawal compared to reducing doses of methadone, alpha$_2$-adrenergic agonists, symptomatic medications or placebo, or in comparison with different buprenorphine regimes. *Other outcomes*: Withdrawal signs and symptoms, completion of withdrawal and adverse effects.

Study population: Subjects primarily opioid dependent and underwent managed withdrawal.

Alcohol and Drug Misuse: A Cochrane Handbook, First Edition. Iosief Abraha and Cristina Cusi.
© 2012 John Wiley & Sons, Ltd. Published 2012 by John Wiley & Sons, Ltd.

Search strategy: The Cochrane Central Register of Controlled Trials, *The Cochrane Library* (Issue 3, 2008), MEDLINE (July 2008), EMBASE, PsycINFO (August 2008) and reference lists of articles.

Results: Twenty-two randomised trials with 1736 participants were included.
- *Buprenorphine versus methadone (five studies)*: Severity of withdrawal, withdrawal symptoms and completion of withdrawal treatment were similar for both medications.
- *Buprenorphine versus clonidine or lofexidine (12 studies)*: Patients treated with buprenorphine had ameliorated the symptoms of withdrawal, stayed in treatment for longer (SMD 0.92, 95% CI 0.57 to 1.27, P < 0.001), and were more likely to complete withdrawal treatment (RR 1.64; 95% CI 1.31–2.06, P < 0.001). No significant differences in the incidence of adverse effects were observed in the two regimens.

What this review adds to the current knowledge: Buprenorphine and methadone in tapered doses appear to have similar efficacy in the management of opioid withdrawal, but withdrawal symptoms may resolve more quickly with buprenorphine.

Buprenorphine is more effective than clonidine or lofexidine in reducing the signs and symptoms of opioid withdrawal, retaining patients in withdrawal treatment and supporting the completion of withdrawal. Buprenorphine may be associated with less drop-out due to adverse effects. This finding holds for both inpatient and outpatient settings, particularly for withdrawal from heroin. The use of buprenorphine to manage withdrawal may also be associated with higher rates of engagement in post-detoxification treatment.

Main limitations: Only a few studies were assessed as having a high risk of allocation and assessment bias. None of the studies were considered at high risk of reporting bias or of incomplete outcome data.

The future: Further research is required to determine the degree of the potential benefit of buprenorphine for management of opioid withdrawal in outpatient settings relative to methadone. Also, the optimum approach to withdrawal following long-term buprenorphine substitution treatment remains unclear.

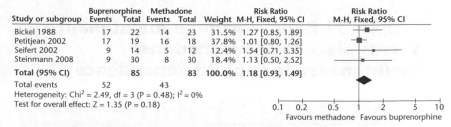

Study or subgroup	Buprenorphine Events	Total	Methadone Events	Total	Weight	Risk Ratio M-H, Fixed, 95% CI
Bickel 1988	17	22	14	23	31.5%	1.27 [0.85, 1.89]
Petitjean 2002	17	19	16	18	37.8%	1.01 [0.80, 1.26]
Seifert 2002	9	14	5	12	12.4%	1.54 [0.71, 3.35]
Steinmann 2008	9	30	8	30	18.4%	1.13 [0.50, 2.52]
Total (95% CI)		85		83	100.0%	1.18 [0.93, 1.49]
Total events	52		43			

Heterogeneity: Chi² = 2.49, df = 3 (P = 0.48); I² = 0%
Test for overall effect: Z = 1.35 (P = 0.18)

Favours methadone   Favours buprenorphine

Figure 38.1 Buprenorphine versus methadone, outcome: completion of withdrawal. Reproduced from Gowing L, Ali R, White JM. Buprenorphine for the management of opioid withdrawal. Cochrane Database Syst Rev. 2009(3):CD002025, with permission from John Wiley & Sons Ltd. Copyright © 2009 The Cochrane Collaboration.

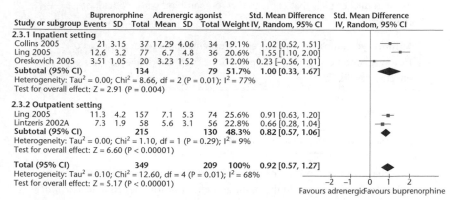

Study or subgroup	Buprenorphine			Adrenergic agonist				Std. Mean Difference IV, Random, 95% CI
	Events	SD	Total	Mean	SD	Total	Weight	
2.3.1 Inpatient setting								
Collins 2005	21	3.15	37	17.29	4.06	34	19.1%	1.02 [0.52, 1.51]
Ling 2005	12.6	3.2	77	6.7	4.8	36	20.6%	1.55 [1.10, 2.00]
Oreskovich 2005	3.51	1.05	20	3.23	1.52	9	12.0%	0.23 [–0.56, 1.01]
Subtotal (95% CI)			134			79	51.7%	1.00 [0.33, 1.67]

Heterogeneity: Tau² = 0.00; Chi² = 8.66, df = 2 (P = 0.01); I² = 77%
Test for overall effect: Z = 2.91 (P = 0.004)

2.3.2 Outpatient setting								
Ling 2005	11.3	4.2	157	7.1	5.3	74	25.6%	0.91 [0.63, 1.20]
Lintzeris 2002A	7.3	1.9	58	5.6	3.1	56	22.8%	0.66 [0.28, 1.04]
Subtotal (95% CI)			215			130	48.3%	0.82 [0.57, 1.06]

Heterogeneity: Tau² = 0.00; Chi² = 1.10, df = 1 (P = 0.29); I² = 9%
Test for overall effect: Z = 6.60 (P < 0.00001)

| Total (95% CI) | | | 349 | | | 209 | 100% | 0.92 [0.57, 1.27] |

Heterogeneity: Tau² = 0.10; Chi² = 12.60, df = 4 (P = 0.01); I² = 68%
Test for overall effect: Z = 5.17 (P < 0.00001)

Favours adrenergic Favours buprenorphine

Figure 38.2 Buprenorphine versus clonidine, outcome: mean days in treatment. Reproduced from Gowing L, Ali R, White JM. Buprenorphine for the management of opioid withdrawal. Cochrane Database Syst Rev. 2009(3):CD002025, with permission from John Wiley & Sons Ltd. Copyright © 2009 The Cochrane Collaboration.

Reference

1 Gowing L, Ali R, White JM. Buprenorphine for the management of opioid withdrawal. Cochrane Database Syst Rev. 2009(3):CD002025. Epub 2009/07/10.

Chapter 39 **Buprenorphine maintenance versus placebo or methadone maintenance for opioid dependence**[1]

Review question: Is buprenorphine maintenance better than placebo or methadone maintenance for the treatment of opioid dependence?

What is known of this topic: Clinical trials have documented the effectiveness of buprenorphine over placebo medication. There is variation in the results of trials that compared buprenorphine with methadone maintenance.

Summary: Compared with placebo, buprenorphine reduced heroin use. However, when compared with methadone, buprenorphine had less effective results.

Last assessment date: 5 December 2007

Objectives: To assess buprenorphine maintenance compared to placebo and methadone maintenance in the management of opioid dependence. *Primary outcomes*: Retention in treatment, use of opioids and other substance use, criminal activity and mortality. *Other outcomes*: Physical health, psychological health and side effects.

Study population: Opioid-dependent participants.

Search strategy: The Cochrane Drugs and Alcohol Review Group Register, the Cochrane Controlled Trials Register, MEDLINE, EMBASE, Current Contents, Psychlit, CORK, Alcohol and Drug Council of Australia, Australian Drug Foundation, Centre for Education and Information on Drugs and Alcohol, Library of Congress databases and reference lists of identified studies and reviews (October 2006).

Alcohol and Drug Misuse: A Cochrane Handbook, First Edition. Iosief Abraha and Cristina Cusi.
© 2012 John Wiley & Sons, Ltd. Published 2012 by John Wiley & Sons, Ltd.

Results: Twenty-four studies with 4497 participants were included.

- *Buprenorphine versus placebo*: Buprenorphine was significantly superior to placebo in retention of patients in treatment at low doses (five studies with 1131 participants; RR 1.5, 95% CI 1.19–1.88), medium doses (four studies with 887 participants; RR 1.74, 95% CI 1.06–2.87) and high doses (four studies with 728 participants; RR 1.74, 95% CI 1.02–2.96).
- *Buprenorphine (flexible doses) versus methadone (flexible doses)*: The double-blind studies showed buprenorphine was significantly less effective than methadone in retaining patients in treatment (five studies with 788 participants; RR 0.83, 95% CI 0.72–0.95), but showed no difference in suppression of opioid use as measured by urinalysis and self-report for those who remained in treatment.
- *Buprenorphine (medium dose) versus methadone (medium dose)*: There was no advantage for buprenorphine over methadone in retention, and medium-dose buprenorphine was inferior in suppression of heroin use based on urinalysis and one study of self-report.

What this review adds to the current knowledge: There are several trials that evaluated the efficacy of buprenorphine in opioid-dependent subjects for the maintenance treatment of heroin dependence. While buprenorphine is more effective than placebo, it is less effective than methadone in retaining patients in treatment.

Main limitations: The majority of the studies (20 of 25) did not clearly describe the method of allocation concealment; only six studies used the double-blind method.

The future: Factors responsible for retention in the first few weeks or months of treatment in buprenorphine versus methadone can be investigated in future studies.

Review: Buprenorphine maintenance versus placebo or methadone maintenance opioid dependence
Comparison: 1 Flexible dose buprenorphine versus flexible dose methadone
Outcome: 1 retention in treatment

Study or subgroup	buprenorphine n/N	methadone n/N	Risk Ratio M-H, Random, 95% CI	Weight	Risk Ratio M-H, Random, 95% CI
1 Double blind flexible dose studies					
Johnson 2000	32/55	40/55		13.4%	0.80 [0.61, 1.05]
Mattick 2003	96/200	120/205		18.0%	0.82 [0.68, 0.99]
Petitjean 2001	15/27	28/31		10.2%	0.62 [0.43, 0.88]
Strain 1994a	47/84	45/80		13.6%	0.99 [0.76, 1.30]
Strain 1994b	13/24	15/27		6.5%	0.98 [0.59, 1.61]
Subtotal (95% CI)	390	398		61.8%	0.83 [0.72, 0.95]
Total events: 203 (buprenorphine), 248 (methadone)					
Heterogeneity: Tau² = 0.00; Chi² = 4.94, df = 4 (P = 0.29); I² = 19%					
Test for overall effect: Z = 2.63 (P = 0.0086)					
2 Open label flexible dose studies					
Fischer 1999	11/29	22/31		6.2%	0.53 [0.32, 0.90]
Lintzeris 2004	38/81	42/77		12.0%	0.86 [0.63, 1.17]
Neri 2005	29/31	28/31		20.0%	1.04 [0.89, 1.20]
Subtotal (95% CI)	141	139		38.2%	0.82 [0.55, 1.23]
Total events: 78 (buprenorphine), 340 (methadone)					
Heterogeneity: Tau² = 0.10; Chi² = 10.80, df = 2 (P = 0.005); I² = 81%					
Test for overall effect: Z = 0.95 (P = 0.34)					
Total (95% CI)	531	537		100.0%	0.85 [0.73, 0.98]
Total events: 203 (buprenorphine), 248 (methadone)					
Heterogeneity: Tau² = 0.02; Chi² = 15.83, df = 7 (P = 0.03); I² = 56%					
Test for overall effect: Z = 2.21 (P = 0.027)					

```
                    0.01    0.1      1      10     100
                      Favours MMT        Favours BMT
```

Figure 39.1 Flexible-dose buprenorphine versus flexible-dose methadone, outcome: retention in treatment. Reproduced from Mattick RP, Kimber J, Breen C, Davoli M. Buprenorphine maintenance versus placebo or methadone maintenance for opioid dependence. Cochrane Database Syst Rev. 2008(2):CD002207, with permission from John Wiley & Sons Ltd. Copyright © 2008 The Cochrane Collaboration.

Reference

1 Mattick RP, Kimber J, Breen C, Davoli M. Buprenorphine maintenance versus placebo or methadone maintenance for opioid dependence. Cochrane Database Syst Rev. 2008(2):CD002207. Epub 2008/04/22.

Chapter 40 Methadone at tapered doses for the management of opioid withdrawal[1]

Review question: What is the effectiveness of tapered methadone's efficacy in managing opioid withdrawal?

What is known of this topic: Dependence on opioid drugs produces major health and social problems. Managed withdrawal, or detoxification, is not in itself a treatment for dependence, but detoxification remains a required first step for many forms of longer term treatment. Despite widespread use, the evidence of tapered methadone's efficacy in managing opioid withdrawal has not been systematically evaluated.

Summary: Tapered methadone compared with other pharmacological treatments showed no substantial clinical difference in terms of completion of treatment, degree of discomfort and results at follow-up, although symptoms experienced by participants differed according to the medication used and the programme adopted.

Last assessment date: 25 March 2008

Objectives: To assess the effectiveness of methadone at tapered doses versus placebo or other pharmacological treatments for the management of detoxification on completion and acceptability of the treatment and relapse rate. *Outcomes considered*: Completion of treatment, acceptability of treatment (duration and severity of signs and symptoms of withdrawal, including patient self-rating), side effects, use of primary substance of abuse, results at follow-up and naloxone challenge.

Study population: Opioid users enrolled in short-term tapered methadone treatment to manage withdrawal from heroin, methadone or buprenorphine (countries of recruitment: United States, United Kingdom, Spain, China, Germany, Italy and Iran).

Search strategy: *The Cochrane Library* (Issue 2, 2008), PubMed, EMBASE, CINAHL, PsycINFO (December 2004) and reference lists of articles.

Alcohol and Drug Misuse: A Cochrane Handbook, First Edition. Iosief Abraha and Cristina Cusi.
© 2012 John Wiley & Sons, Ltd. Published 2012 by John Wiley & Sons, Ltd.

Results: Twenty trials involving 1907 people were included.
- *Methadone versus placebo (two studies)*: Significant completion of treatment rates was observed in the placebo group (RR 1.95, CI 95% 1.21–3.13).
- *Methadone versus any other drug treatment*: There was no clinical difference in terms of completion of treatment (RR 1.08, 95% CI 0.95–1.24) and results at follow-up (RR 1.17, 95% CI 0.72–1.92).

It was not possible to pool data for the other outcomes; however, no significant differences were observed between the considered treatments (tapered methadone versus adrenergic agonists; 11 studies), other opioid agonists (five studies) and anxiolytics (two studies).

What this review adds to the current knowledge: The results indicate that the medications used in the included studies are similar in terms of overall effectiveness. For important outcomes such as withdrawal symptoms, treatment programmes are difficult to compare due to the variability of the methods used to assess them. Withdrawal limited to 30 days has the disadvantage that many persons, due to the rapid tapering, are prematurely withdrawn and consequently resume heroin use.

Main limitations: There was a wide variation in the treatment regimes that hindered the application of meta-analysis for several outcomes.

The future: Randomised trials that use standardised criteria for reporting urinalysis are needed in order to enable comparison and pooling of results.

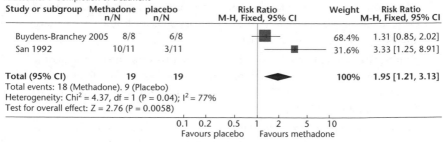

Review: Methadone at tapered doses for the management of opioid withdrawal
Comparison: 5 Tapered methadone versus placebo
Outcome: 1 Completion of treatment

Study or subgroup	Methadone n/N	placebo n/N	Risk Ratio M-H, Fixed, 95% CI	Weight	Risk Ratio M-H, Fixed, 95% CI
Buydens-Branchey 2005	8/8	6/8		68.4%	1.31 [0.85, 2.02]
San 1992	10/11	3/11		31.6%	3.33 [1.25, 8.91]
Total (95% CI)	**19**	**19**		**100%**	**1.95 [1.21, 3.13]**

Total events: 18 (Methadone). 9 (Placebo)
Heterogeneity: Chi^2 = 4.37, df = 1 (P = 0.04); I^2 = 77%
Test for overall effect: Z = 2.76 (P = 0.0058)

0.1   0.2   0.5   1   2   5   10
Favours placebo   Favours methadone

Figure 40.1 Tapered methadone versus placebo, outcome: completion of treatment. Reproduced from Amato L, Davoli M, Minozzi S, Ali R, Ferri M. Methadone at tapered doses for the management of opioid withdrawal. Cochrane Database Syst Rev. 2005(3):CD003409, with permission from John Wiley & Sons Ltd. Copyright © 2005 The Cochrane Collaboration.

Review: Methadone at tapered doses for the management of opiod withdrawal
Comparison: 1 Tapered methadone versus any other treatment
Outcome: 1 Completion of treatment

Study or subgroup	Methadone n/N	Other pharmac treatment n/N	Risk Ratio M-H, Random, 95% CI	Weight	Risk Ratio M-H, Random, 95% CI
Steinmann 2007	6/21	9/18		2.4%	0.57 [0.25, 1.30]
Seifert 2002	5/12	9/14		2.6%	0.65 [0.30, 1.41]
San 1994	31/75	34/69		8.1%	0.84 [0.58, 1.20]
Kleber 1985	21/25	24/24		14.2%	0.84 [0.70, 1.01]
Salehi 2007	22/37	22/35		7.9%	0.95 [0.65, 1.37]
Buydens-Branchey 2005	8/8	21/23		13.2%	1.05 [0.86, 1.30]
Drummond 1989	5/13	4/11		1.5%	1.06 [0.37, 3.00]
Sorensen 1982	5/15	4/13		1.4%	1.08 [0.37, 3.21]
Bearn 1996	43/44	36/42		16.3%	1.14 [1.00, 1.30]
Umbricht 2003	9/18	15/37		3.9%	1.23 [0.67, 2.26]
Howells 2002	28/36	19/32		8.8%	1.31 [0.94, 1.83]
San 1990	30/40	67/130		11.8%	1.46 [1.14, 1.86]
Washton 1981	6/13	4/13		1.6%	1.50 [0.55, 4.10]
Tennant 1975	25/36	15/36		6.2%	1.67 [1.07, 2.60]
Total (95% CI)	**393**	**497**		**100.0%**	**1.08 [0.95, 1.24]**

Total events: 244 (Methadone). 283 (Other pharmac treatment)
Heterogeneity: Tau^2 = 0.02; Chi^2 = 25.36, df = 13 (P = 0.02); I^2 = 49%
Test for overall effect: Z = 1.14 (P = 0.26)

```
          0.001 0.01  0.1    1    10   100  1000
          Favours other ph. tr   Favours methadone
```

Figure 40.2 Tapered methadone versus any other treatment, outcome: completion of treatment. Reproduced from Amato L, Davoli M, Minozzi S, Ali R, Ferri M. Methadone at tapered doses for the management of opioid withdrawal. Cochrane Database Syst Rev. 2005(3):CD003409, with permission from John Wiley & Sons Ltd. Copyright © 2005 The Cochrane Collaboration.

Reference

1 Amato L, Davoli M, Minozzi S, Ali R, Ferri M. Methadone at tapered doses for the management of opioid withdrawal. Cochrane Database Syst Rev. 2005 (3):CD003409. Epub 2005/07/22.

Chapter 41 **Methadone maintenance at different dosages for opioid dependence**[1]

Review question: What is the appropriate dosage of methadone effective in retaining patients and in reducing use of heroin and cocaine for opioid-dependent patients?

What is known of this topic: Methadone maintenance treatment is a long-term opioid replacement therapy that is effective in the management of opioid dependence. Although methadone is recommended at high dosages for reducing illicit opioid use and promoting longer retention in treatment, current dosage of methadone as a maintenance therapy varies widely.

Summary: Methadone dosages ranging from 60 to 100 mg/day are more effective than lower dosages in retaining patients and in reducing use of heroin and cocaine during treatment.

Last assessment date: 1 May 2003

Objectives: To evaluate the efficacy and safety of different dosages of methadone maintenance treatment for opioid dependence, in modifying health and social outcomes and in promoting patients' familial, occupational and relational functioning.

Study population: Opioid-dependent patients (studies on pregnant women were excluded).

Search strategy: Medline, EMBASE, ERIC, PsycINFO, Cochrane Controlled Trials Register and Register of the Cochrane Drugs and Alcohol Group (2001).

Results: Eleven randomised clinical trials with 2279 participants and 10 controlled prospective studies with 3715 participants were included.

Alcohol and Drug Misuse: A Cochrane Handbook, First Edition. Iosief Abraha and Cristina Cusi.
© 2012 John Wiley & Sons, Ltd. Published 2012 by John Wiley & Sons, Ltd.

Randomised trials: The retention rate was significantly elevated in the high-dose group, both at shorter follow-ups (RR 1.36, 1.13–1.63) and at longer ones (RR 1.62, 0.95–2.77), compared to the low-dose group.

The use of opioids (self-reported) was significantly lower in the high-dose group than in the middle-dose group (WMD −1.89, −3.43 to −0.35) and in the low-dose group (WMD −2.00, −4.77 to 0.77).

The rate of opioid abstinence, (urine based at >3–4 weeks) was significantly better in the high-dose group than in the low-dose groups (RR 1.59, 1.16–2.18) and the middle-dose group (RR 1.5, 0.63–3.61).

The rate of cocaine abstinence (urine based at >3–4 weeks) was significantly better in the high-dose group than in the low-dose group (RR 1.81, 1.15–2.85).

Controlled prospective studies: Mortality rate was not significantly different between the comparisons: high dose versus low dose at 6 years follow-up (RR 0.29, 0.02–5.34), high dose versus middle dose at 6 years follow-up (RR 0.38, 0.02–9.34) and middle dose versus low dose at 6 years follow-up (RR 0.57, 0.06–5.06).

What this review adds to the current knowledge: Methadone dosages ranging from 60 to 100 mg/day had more effective results than lower dosages in retaining patients and in reducing use of heroin and cocaine during treatment.

Main limitations: The allocation method of the 11 randomised trials was not clearly described. Heterogeneity and outcome reporting bias are potential threats to the validity of the results of the current review.

The future: The last update of the review dates back to 2003, therefore future research may change the current conclusions. Future trials should overcome the present methodological problems (including the heterogeneity of outcome indicators) and should address the effect of methadone dose in mortality reduction.

Reference

1 Faggiano F, Vigna-Taglianti F, Versino E, Lemma P. Methadone maintenance at different dosages for opioid dependence. Cochrane Database Syst Rev. 2003(3):CD002208.

Chapter 42 **Methadone maintenance therapy versus no opioid replacement therapy for opioid dependence**[1]

Review question: Is methadone maintenance treatment for opioid dependence effective compared to treatments that do not include opioid replacement therapy?

What is known of this topic: Methadone maintenance treatment remains one of the best researched treatments for opioid dependence. It is effective in reducing illicit opiate use compared to no treatment, drug-free treatment, placebo or detoxification. Trials have been conducted in different countries and treatment settings.

Summary answer: Methadone is an effective maintenance therapy for the treatment of heroin dependence. It retains patients in treatment and decreases heroin use better than treatments that do not utilise opioid replacement therapy.

Last assessment date: 18 February 2009

Objectives: To evaluate the effectiveness of methadone maintenance treatment on opioid dependence compared with treatments that did not include an opioid replacement therapy. *Primary outcomes*: Retention in treatment, mortality, proportion of urine or hair analysis results positive for heroin (or morphine), self-reported heroin use and criminal activity. *Other outcomes*: Use of other drugs, physical health and psychological health.

Study population: Opioid-dependent individuals.

Search strategy: The Cochrane Controlled Trials Register, EMBASE, PubMed, CINAHL, Current Contents, Psychlit, CORK, Alcohol and Drug Council of Australia, Australian Drug Foundation, Centre for Education and Information on Drugs and Alcohol, Australian Bibliographic Network, Library of

---

Alcohol and Drug Misuse: A Cochrane Handbook, First Edition. Iosief Abraha and Cristina Cusi.
© 2012 John Wiley & Sons, Ltd. Published 2012 by John Wiley & Sons, Ltd.

Congress databases, available NIDA monographs and the College on Problems of Drug Dependence Inc. (December 2008).

Results: Eleven randomised trials with 1969 participants were included.

- *Methadone maintenance treatment versus no methadone maintenance treatment – retention in treatment (seven studies):* Results from all studies showed that methadone was superior in retention rate; however, there was significant heterogeneity within studies. Subgroup analyses: pooled results from older studies (pre-2000) were in favour of methadone (three studies with 505 patients; RR 0.33, 95% CI 0.19–0.57, heterogeneity $I^2 = 75\%$, P = 0.02); pooled results from recent studies were also in favour of methadone (four studies with 750 patients; RR 4.44, 95%CI 3.26–2.04, no significant heterogeneity).

Methadone was also superior in terms of suppression of heroin use based on urine and hair samples (six studies with 1129 patients; RR 0.66, 95% CI 0.56–0.78). There was no significant difference in terms of criminal activity (three randomised trials; RR 0.39, 95% CI 0.12–1.25) and mortality (four trials; RR 0.48, 95% CI 0.10–2.39) between the two comparisons.

What this review adds to the current knowledge: Several randomised trials that tested the efficacy of methadone maintenance therapy for the management of opioid dependence were published. Methadone maintenance treatment is able to retain patients in treatment, and suppress heroin, better than the drug-free alternatives (placebo medication, offer of drug-free treatment, detoxification or wait-list control), and in patient self-report.

Main limitations: There was a considerable heterogeneity within studies, although sub-analyses showed consistent findings in favour of methadone maintenance treatment.

The future: There is no need to conduct further randomised trials on the effectiveness of methadone as a maintenance therapy. However, evidence on reduction of criminal activity and mortality needs to be addressed from studies including observational trials.

Review: Methadone maintenance therapy versus no opioid replacement therapy for opioid dependence
Comparison: 1 Methadone maintenance treatment vs No methadone maintenance treatment
Outcome: 1 Retention in treatment

Study or subgroup	Methadone MT n/N	Control n/N	Risk Ratio M-H, Random, 95% CI	Weight	Risk Ratio M-H, Random, 95% CI
1 Old studies (pre 2000)					
Newman 1979	38/50	5/50		22.2%	7.60 [3.26, 17.71]
Strain 1993a	44/84	17/81		35.2%	2.50 [1.56, 3.99]
Vanichseni 1991	91/120	41/120		42.6%	2.22 [1.70, 2.90]
Subtotal (95% CI)	**254**	**251**		**100.0%**	**3.05 [1.75, 5.35]**
Total events: 173 (Methadone MT), 63 (Control)					
Heterogeneity: Tau^2 = 0.17; Chi^2 = 8.01, df = 2 (P = 0.02); I^2 = 75%					
Test for overall effect: Z = 3.91 (P = 0.000092)					
2 New studies					
Gruber 2008	46/72	4/39		16.7%	6.23 [2.42, 16.02]
Kinlock 2007	43/71	5/70		18.4%	8.48 [3.57, 20.14]
Schwartz 2006	151/199	25/120		33.5%	3.64 [2.55, 5.21]
Sees 2000	78/91	18/88		31.5%	4.19 [2.75, 6.38]
Subtotal (95% CI)	**433**	**317**		**100.0%**	**4.44 [3.26, 6.04]**
Total events: 318 (Methadone MT), 52 (Control)					
Heterogeneity: Tau^2 = 0.02; Chi^2 = 3.09, df = 3 (P = 0.27); I^2 = 23%					
Test for overall effect: Z = 9.48 (P < 0.00001)					

```
        0.002    0.1      1      10     500
        Favours control       Favours Methadone
```

Figure 42.1 Methadone maintenance treatment versus no methadone maintenance treatment, outcome: retention in treatment. Reproduced from Mattick RP, Breen C, Kimber J, Davoli M. Methadone maintenance therapy versus no opioid replacement therapy for opioid dependence. Cochrane Database Syst Rev. 2009(3):CD002209, with permission from John Wiley & Sons Ltd. Copyright © 2009 The Cochrane Collaboration.

Reference

1 Mattick RP, Breen C, Kimber J, Davoli M. Methadone maintenance therapy versus no opioid replacement therapy for opioid dependence. Cochrane Database Syst Rev. 2009(3):CD002209.

Chapter 43 **Opioid antagonists under heavy sedation or anaesthesia for opioid withdrawal**[1]

Review question: Is the administration of opioid antagonists under heavy sedation or anaesthesia an effective approach to the management of opioid withdrawal?

What is known of this topic: People who are opioid dependent find it difficult to complete detoxification. The use of opioid antagonists to induce withdrawal in conjunction with heavy sedation or anaesthesia to remove the experience of withdrawal symptoms has been proposed to accelerate detoxification. However, controversy exists about the administration of opioid antagonists either because its use has been promoted without evidence of efficacy or because it may expose patients to potentially life-threatening risks (including aspiration pneumonia and cardiac arrhythmias).

Summary: Antagonist-induced withdrawal under heavy sedation or anaesthesia cannot be supported due to the potentially life-threatening nature of the adverse events.

Last assessment date: 16 August 2009

Objectives: To assess the effectiveness of opioid antagonists to induce opioid withdrawal with concomitant heavy sedation or anaesthesia. *Outcomes considered*: Intensity and duration of withdrawal signs and symptoms, duration of withdrawal treatment, completion of treatment and occurrence of adverse events.

Study population: Participants who were primarily opioid dependent and underwent managed withdrawal.

Alcohol and Drug Misuse: A Cochrane Handbook, First Edition. Iosief Abraha and Cristina Cusi.
© 2012 John Wiley & Sons, Ltd. Published 2012 by John Wiley & Sons, Ltd.

Search strategy: *The Cochrane Library* (Issue 3, 2009), MEDLINE (August 2009), EMBASE (Week 32, 2009), PsycINFO (July 2009) and reference lists of articles.

Results: Nine studies (eight randomised trials) involving 1109 participants were included.

Antagonist-induced withdrawal is more intense but less prolonged than withdrawal managed with reducing doses of methadone, and doses of naltrexone sufficient for blockade of opioid effects can be established significantly more quickly with antagonist-induced withdrawal than withdrawal managed with clonidine and symptomatic medications. The level of sedation does not affect the intensity and duration of withdrawal, although the duration of anaesthesia may influence withdrawal severity. There is a significantly greater risk of adverse events with heavy, compared to light, sedation (RR 3.21, 95% CI 1.13–9.12, P = 0.03) and probably with this approach compared to other forms of detoxification.

What this review adds to the current knowledge: The intensity of withdrawal experienced with anaesthesia-based approaches is similar to that experienced with approaches using only minimal sedation, but there is a significantly increased risk of serious adverse events with anaesthesia-assisted approaches. The lack of additional benefit, and increased risk of harm, suggest that this form of treatment should not be pursued.

Main limitations: The risk of allocation bias was judged high in only two studies. Outcome reporting bias cannot be excluded.

The future: Research resources should be directed towards assessment and development of minimal sedation approaches, or the use of buprenorphine to facilitate transition to naltrexone maintenance treatment.

Reference

1 Gowing L, Ali R, White JM. Opioid antagonists under heavy sedation or anaesthesia for opioid withdrawal. Cochrane Database Syst Rev. 2010(1):CD002022.

Chapter 44 Opioid antagonists with minimal sedation for opioid withdrawal[1]

Review question: Are opioid antagonists in combination with minimal sedation effective for the management of opioid withdrawal?

What is known of this topic: The rationale underlying the use of opioid antagonists to induce withdrawal is that a more rapid transition from dependence to abstinence might increase rates of completion of withdrawal. In this approach, adjunct medications (clonidine or lofexidine, for light sedation) are used to reduce the severity of withdrawal experienced after administration of opioid antagonists.

Summary: Although the use of opioid antagonists combined with alpha$_2$-adrenergic agonists is a feasible approach to the management of opioid withdrawal, evidence on the effectiveness of the approach is of low quality, leaving uncertainty about its value.

Last assessment date: 14 January 2009

Objectives: To assess the effectiveness of opioid antagonists in combination with minimal sedation to manage opioid withdrawal. *Primary outcomes*: Intensity of withdrawal, duration of treatment, nature and incidence of adverse effects and completion of treatment. *Other outcomes*: Number of participants engaged in further treatment following completion of the withdrawal intervention.

Study population: Participants who were primarily opioid dependent and underwent managed withdrawal.

Search strategy: *The Cochrane Library* (Issue 3, 2008), MEDLINE (July 2008), EMBASE (Week 31, 2008), PsycINFO (August 2008) and reference lists of articles.

Alcohol and Drug Misuse: A Cochrane Handbook, First Edition. Iosief Abraha and Cristina Cusi.
© 2012 John Wiley & Sons, Ltd. Published 2012 by John Wiley & Sons, Ltd.

Results: Nine studies (six randomised trials) with 837 participants were included.

Overall, results suggested that withdrawal induced by opioid antagonists in combination with an adrenergic agonist is more intense than withdrawal managed with clonidine or lofexidine alone, but the overall severity is less. Delirium may occur following the first dose of opioid antagonist, particularly with higher doses (>25 mg naltrexone). However, the quality of the evidence was low.

In some situations, antagonist-induced withdrawal may be associated with significantly higher rates of completion of treatment, compared to withdrawal managed primarily with adrenergic agonists. However, this outcome has not been produced consistently, and the extent of any benefit is highly uncertain.

What this review adds to the current knowledge: Although several publications were present in the medical literature and the results suggested that the use of opioid antagonists in combination with minimal sedation is a feasible approach to the management of opioid withdrawal, the lack of studies with a low risk of bias and the heterogeneity in study design and findings make any conclusions highly uncertain.

Main limitations: Heterogeneity and the absence of studies with low risk of bias.

The future: Research should be of high methodological quality and more consistent in outcome measures. Comparisons that include withdrawal from methadone are also required with assessment of both objective and subjective signs and symptoms of withdrawal as well as side effects of treatment (delirium, hypotension, sedation and dry mouth). Antagonist-induced withdrawal approaches should also be compared with approaches based on buprenorphine.

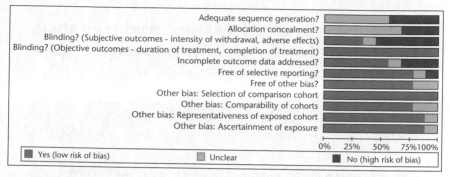

Figure 44.1 Methodological quality graph: review authors' judgements about each methodological quality item presented as percentages across all included studies. Reproduced from Gowing L, Ali R, White JM. Opioid antagonists with minimal sedation for opioid withdrawal. Cochrane Database Syst Rev. 2009 (4):CD002021, with permission from John Wiley & Sons Ltd. Copyright © 2009 The Cochrane Collaboration.

Reference

1 Gowing L, Ali R, White JM. Opioid antagonists with minimal sedation for opioid withdrawal. Cochrane Database Syst Rev. 2009(4):CD002021.

Chapter 45 **Oral naltrexone maintenance treatment for opioid dependence**[1]

Review question: Is naltrexone as a maintenance treatment better than placebo or other treatments in preventing relapse in opioid addicts after detoxification?

What is known of this topic: Naltrexone is an opioid antagonist that has no euphoric effects and could provide a non-addicting treatment for opioid users. There are selected patient groups who may be good candidates for naltrexone treatment (e.g. health professionals, business executives and individuals under legal supervision). Sustained-release preparations that reduce the frequency of dosing may make naltrexone an alternative effective treatment.

Summary: Naltrexone did not provide any advantage over no treatment or psychotherapy in preventing relapse after detoxification.

Last assessment date: 3 January 2011

Objectives: To evaluate the effects of naltrexone maintenance treatment with respect to placebo or other treatments in preventing relapse in opioid addicts after detoxification. *Primary outcomes*: Retention and abstinence, abstinence at follow-up and mortality. *Other outcomes*: Side effects and criminal activity.

Study population: Participants dependent on heroin, or former heroin addicts dependent on methadone and participating in a naltrexone treatment programme are considered.

Search strategy: *The Cochrane Library* (Issue 6, 2010), PubMed and CINAHL (June 2010). Also inspected reference lists of relevant articles and contacted pharmaceutical producers of naltrexone, authors and other Cochrane Review groups.

Alcohol and Drug Misuse: A Cochrane Handbook, First Edition. Iosief Abraha and Cristina Cusi.
© 2012 John Wiley & Sons, Ltd. Published 2012 by John Wiley & Sons, Ltd.

Results: Thirteen studies with 1158 participants were included.

• *Naltrexone alone or associated with psychosocial therapy versus placebo or no treatment*: For the outcomes retention in treatment and abstinence during the study and abstinence at follow-up, a naltrexone-based regimen was not effective.

No significant difference was found in terms of side effects between the different regimens.

With respect to the number of participants re-incarcerated during the study period, naltrexone had more effective results than placebo or no pharmacological treatment (RR 0.47, 95% CI 0.26–0.84).

Naltrexone was not superior to benzodiazepines or to buprenorphine for retention and abstinence and side effects. Results come from single studies.

What this review adds to the current knowledge: Although several studies have examined the efficacy of naltrexone, it did not provide any advantage as a maintenance treatment for retention in treatment and abstinence and for abstinence at follow-up.

Main limitations: Few trials reported adequate sequence generation and allocation concealment. Attrition bias was not of concern to the validity of the results.

The future: Randomised trials evaluating effectiveness for treatment of opioid dependence should compare oral naltrexone to sustained-release naltrexone or agonist replacement treatment with methadone or buprenorphine. Research on naltrexone should also focus on mortality and other safety outcomes to make a harm–benefit analysis possible.

Review: Oral naltrexone maintenance treatment for opioid dependence
Comparison: 1 naltrexone versus placebo or no pharmacological treatments
Outcome: 2 retention and abstinence, all patients

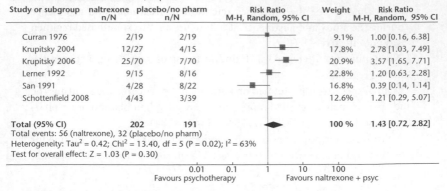

Study or subgroup	naltrexone n/N	placebo/no pharm n/N	Risk Ratio M-H, Random, 95% CI	Weight	Risk Ratio M-H, Random, 95% CI
Curran 1976	2/19	2/19		9.1%	1.00 [0.16, 6.38]
Krupitsky 2004	12/27	4/15		17.8%	2.78 [1.03, 7.49]
Krupitsky 2006	25/70	7/70		20.9%	3.57 [1.65, 7.71]
Lerner 1992	9/15	8/16		22.8%	1.20 [0.63, 2.28]
San 1991	4/28	8/22		16.8%	0.39 [0.14, 1.14]
Schottenfield 2008	4/43	3/39		12.6%	1.21 [0.29, 5.07]
Total (95% CI)	202	191		100 %	1.43 [0.72, 2.82]

Total events: 56 (naltrexone), 32 (placebo/no pharm)
Heterogeneity: Tau^2 = 0.42; Chi^2 = 13.40, df = 5 (P = 0.02); I^2 = 63%
Test for overall effect: Z = 1.03 (P = 0.30)

0.01   0.1   1   10   100
Favours psychotherapy   Favours naltrexone + psyc

Figure 45.1 Naltrexone versus placebo or no pharmacological treatments, outcome: retention and abstinence in all patients. Reproduced from Minozzi S, Amato L, Vecchi S, Davoli M, Kirchmayer U, Verster A. Oral naltrexone maintenance treatment for opioid dependence. Cochrane Database Syst Rev. 2011(2):CD001333, with permission from John Wiley & Sons Ltd. Copyright © 2011 The Cochrane Collaboration.

Review: Oral naltrexone maintenance treatment for opioid dependence
Comparison: 1 naltrexone versus placebo or no pharmacological treatments
Outcome: 3 retention and abstinence, patients forced to abstinence

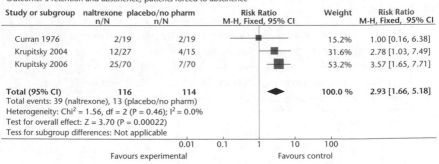

Study or subgroup	naltrexone n/N	placebo/no pharm n/N	Risk Ratio M-H, Fixed, 95% CI	Weight	Risk Ratio M-H, Fixed, 95% CI
Curran 1976	2/19	2/19		15.2%	1.00 [0.16, 6.38]
Krupitsky 2004	12/27	4/15		31.6%	2.78 [1.03, 7.49]
Krupitsky 2006	25/70	7/70		53.2%	3.57 [1.65, 7.71]
Total (95% CI)	116	114		100.0 %	2.93 [1.66, 5.18]

Total events: 39 (naltrexone), 13 (placebo/no pharm)
Heterogeneity: Chi^2 = 1.56, df = 2 (P = 0.46); I^2 = 0.0%
Test for overall effect: Z = 3.70 (P = 0.00022)
Tess for subgroup differences: Not applicable

0.01   0.1   1   10   100
Favours experimental   Favours control

Figure 45.2 Naltrexone versus placebo or no pharmacological treatments, outcome: retention and abstinence in patients forced to abstinence. Reproduced from Minozzi S, Amato L, Vecchi S, Davoli M, Kirchmayer U, Verster A. Oral naltrexone maintenance treatment for opioid dependence. Cochrane Database Syst Rev. 2011(2):CD001333, with permission from John Wiley & Sons Ltd. Copyright © 2011 The Cochrane Collaboration.

Reference

1 Minozzi S, Amato L, Vecchi S, Davoli M, Kirchmayer U, Verster A. Oral naltrexone maintenance treatment for opioid dependence. Cochrane Database Syst Rev. 2011(2):CD001333.

Chapter 46 **Sustained-release naltrexone for opioid dependence**[1]

Review question: Is sustained-release naltrexone effective for opioid dependence?

What is known of this topic: Opioid dependence is a chronic lifelong relapsing disorder, which requires substantial therapeutic efforts to keep patients drug free. Methadone is currently the most effective and well-investigated treatment for opioid dependence. Naltrexone is an opioid antagonist which effectively blocks heroin effects. Since the use of naltrexone tablets is associated with high drop-out rates, several depot injections and implants can be a valid alternative.

Summary: There is insufficient evidence to conclude that sustained-release naltrexone is effective for opioid dependence.

Last assessment date: 24 January 2008

Objectives: To evaluate the effect of sustained-release naltrexone for opioid dependence compared to placebo or alternative treatment. *Primary outcomes*: Opioid use during and after treatment, treatment adherence, induction, compliance with protocol, retention in treatment and adverse effects. *Other outcomes*: Use of other illicit drugs, criminal activity and incarceration, quality of life, mental health and duration of achieved therapeutic naltrexone blood levels.

Study population: Adults or adolescents with opioid dependence. For safety assessment, other alcohol-dependent samples were also considered.

Search strategy: The Cochrane Central Register of Controlled Trials, MEDLINE, EMBASE, CINAHL, LILACS, PsycINFO, ISI Web of Science, trial database at http://clinicaltrials.gov, available NIDA monographs and CPDD and AAAP conference proceedings (November 2007).

Alcohol and Drug Misuse: A Cochrane Handbook, First Edition. Iosief Abraha and Cristina Cusi.
© 2012 John Wiley & Sons, Ltd. Published 2012 by John Wiley & Sons, Ltd.

Results: Seventeen studies were included.

For effectiveness, one randomised trial met inclusion criteria (60 participants). Two dosages of naltrexone depot injections (192 and 384 mg) were compared to placebo. High-dose significantly increased days in treatment compared to placebo (WMD 21.00, 95% CI 10.68 to 31.32). High-dose compared to low-dose significantly increased days in treatment (WMD 12.00, 95% CI 1.69 to 22.31, P = 0.02). Number of patients retained in treatment did not show significant differences between groups.

For adverse effects, 17 reports met inclusion criteria analyses, and six were randomised trials. Side effects were significantly more frequent in naltrexone depot groups compared to placebo. In alcohol-dependent samples only, adverse effects appeared to be significantly more frequent in the low-dose naltrexone depot groups compared to placebo (RR 1.18, 95% CI 1.02–1.36, P = 0.02). In the opioid-dependent sample, group differences were not statistically significant. Reports on systematic assessment of side effects and adverse events were scarce.

What this review adds to the current knowledge: The naltrexone depot injection appeared dose-dependently beneficial for opioid dependence. Adverse effects were significantly more frequent in the naltrexone group. Evidence was scarce since only one randomised trial with a limited number of participants addressed the effectiveness of naltrexone.

Main limitations: Only one randomised trial with limited number of participants addressed the effectiveness of naltrexone. No direct comparison was made with methadone.

The future: Future studies of sustained-release naltrexone involving opioid-dependent patients should be randomised, provide a complete description of drop-out and be compared with methadone maintenance or another treatment.

Reference

1 Lobmaier P, Kornor H, Kunoe N, Bjorndal A. Sustained-release naltrexone for opioid dependence. Cochrane Database Syst Rev. 2008(2):CD006140.

Chapter 47 **Heroin maintenance for chronic heroin-dependent individuals**[1]

Review question: Is prescription of heroin to heroin-dependent subjects effective for maintenance therapy?

What is known of this topic: Several approaches are used to stabilise heroin users including methadone, buprenorphine and methadol. Some experiences suggest that programmes of heroin administration may achieve the reduction of illicit substance use disorders and criminal offences, and achieve stabilisation and the reintegration into the social community. A review is needed to systematically address the issue of heroin maintenance.

Summary: The available evidence suggests an added value of heroin prescribed alongside flexible doses of methadone for long-term, treatment-refractory, opioid users, to reach a decrease in the use of illicit substances, involvement in criminal activity and incarceration, a possible reduction in mortality and an increase in retention in treatment.

Last assessment date: 5 January 2011

Objectives: To compare heroin maintenance to methadone or other substitution treatments for opioid dependence regarding efficacy and acceptability, retaining patients in treatment, reducing the use of illicit substances and improving health and social functioning.

Study population: Adult patients chronically dependent on heroin.

Search strategy: *The Cochrane Library* (Issue 1, 2005), MEDLINE (November 2009), EMBASE (2005) and CINAHL (2005). Personal communications with researchers in the field of heroin prescription identified on-going trials.

Results: Eight studies involving 2007 patients were included.

Five studies compared supervised injected heroin plus flexible dosages of methadone treatment to oral methadone only and showed that heroin helps

Alcohol and Drug Misuse: A Cochrane Handbook, First Edition. Iosief Abraha and Cristina Cusi.
© 2012 John Wiley & Sons, Ltd. Published 2012 by John Wiley & Sons, Ltd.

patients to remain in treatment (valid data from four studies with 1388 participants; RR 1.44, 95% CI 1.19–1.75, heterogeneity P = 0.03), and to reduce use of illicit drugs.

Maintenance with supervised injected heroin has a not statistically significant protective effect on mortality (four studies with 1477 participants; RR 0.65, 95% CI 0.25–1.69, heterogeneity P = 0.89), but it exposes a greater risk of adverse events related to study medication.

Results on criminal activity and incarceration were not possible to be pooled but where the outcomes were measured, results of single studies do provide evidence that heroin provision can reduce criminal activity and incarceration or imprisonment.

Social functioning improved in all the intervention groups with heroin groups having slightly better results. If all the studies comparing heroin provision in any conditions versus any other treatment are pooled, the direction of effect remains in favour of heroin.

What this review adds to the current knowledge: The available evidence suggests an added value of heroin prescribed alongside flexible doses of methadone for long-term, treatment-refractory opioid users, to reach a decrease in the use of illicit substances, a decrease in involvement in criminal activity and incarceration, a possible reduction in mortality and an increase in retention in treatment. Due to the higher rate of serious adverse events, heroin prescription should remain a treatment for people who are currently or have in the past failed maintenance treatment, and it should be provided in clinical settings where proper follow-up is ensured.

Main limitations: Significant heterogeneity was present within the trials that evaluated the outcome retention of treatment.

The future: Heroin provision is now currently provided in several countries. Future randomised trials may provide additional information.

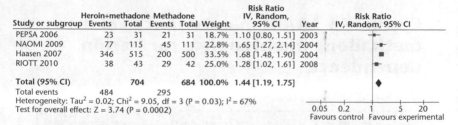

Study or subgroup	Heroin+methadone		Methadone			Risk Ratio IV, Random, 95% CI		Risk Ratio IV, Random, 95% CI
	Events	Total	Events	Total	Weight	95% CI	Year	
PEPSA 2006	23	31	21	31	18.7%	1.10 [0.80, 1.51]	2003	
NAOMI 2009	77	115	45	111	22.8%	1.65 [1.27, 2.14]	2004	
Haasen 2007	346	515	200	500	33.5%	1.68 [1.48, 1.90]	2004	
RIOTT 2010	38	43	29	42	25.0%	1.28 [1.02, 1.61]	2008	
Total (95% CI)		704		684	100.0%	1.44 [1.19, 1.75]		
Total events	484		295					

Heterogeneity: Tau^2 = 0.02; Chi^2 = 9.05, df = 3 (P = 0.03); I^2 = 67%
Test for overall effect: Z = 3.74 (P = 0.0002)

0.05 0.2 1 5 20
Favours control Favours experimental

Figure 47.1 Supervised injected heroin and methadone versus oral methadone. Reproduced from Ferri M, Davoli M, Perucci CA. Heroin maintenance for chronic heroin-dependent individuals. Cochrane Database Syst Rev. 2010(8):CD003410, with permission from John Wiley & Sons Ltd. Copyright © 2010 The Cochrane Collaboration.

Reference

1 Ferri M, Davoli M, Perucci CA. Heroin maintenance for chronic heroin-dependent individuals. Cochrane Database Syst Rev. 2010(8):CD003410. Epub 2010/08/06.

Chapter 48 **LAAM maintenance versus methadone maintenance for heroin dependence**[1]

Review question: Is levo-alpha-acetylmethadol (LAAM) maintenance more effective than methadone maintenance in the treatment of heroin dependence?

What is known of this topic: LAAM is an opiate agonist and has been shown to reduce dependence on heroin when given continuously under supervised dosing conditions. LAAM has a long duration of action requiring dosing every 2 or 3 days compared to methadone which requires daily dosing. LAAM is at risk of being withdrawn from the market following 10 cases of life-threatening cardiac arrhythmias and an association with QT prolongation.

Summary: Although LAAM appears to be more effective than methadone at reducing heroin use, more LAAM-allocated patients ceased their medication during the studies and experienced adverse effects, some of which may be life threatening.

Last assessment date: 4 February 2002

Objectives: To compare the efficacy and acceptability of LAAM maintenance to methadone maintenance in the treatment of heroin dependence in terms of retention in treatment, reduction in opiate use, continuous abstinence from opiates and global assessments of health. *Other outcomes*: All cause mortality, reasons for cessation of treatment, drop-out due to side effects and drop-out due to medication not holding.

Study population: Inpatient or outpatient, heroin dependent or in opioid replacement therapy for heroin-dependent participants.

Alcohol and Drug Misuse: A Cochrane Handbook, First Edition. Iosief Abraha and Cristina Cusi.
© 2012 John Wiley & Sons, Ltd. Published 2012 by John Wiley & Sons, Ltd.

Search strategy: MEDLINE (January 1966–August 2000), PsycINFO (1887–August 2000), EMBASE (January 1985–August 2000), Cochrane Controlled Trials Register (Issue 2, 2000), hand searching of NIDA monographs and reference lists of articles (August 2000) and the Cochrane Group on Drugs and Alcohol's specialised register of trials (February 2003).

Results: Eighteen studies (15 randomised trials with three controlled prospective studies) were included.

- *LAAM versus methadone (11 studies with 1473 participants)*: Treatment cessation was significantly higher in the LAAM group (RR 1.36, 95% CI 1.07–1.73). Non-abstinence was less with LAAM (five studies with 983 participants; RR 0.81, 95% CI 0.72–0.91).

There was a non-significant trend for mortality to be higher with LAAM (two studies with 1441 participants; RR 2.28, 95% CI 0.59–8.90, P = 0.2).

There were almost twice as many drop-outs due to side effects with LAAM than with methadone (two studies with 209 participants; RR 1.88, 95% CI 1.08–3.27, P = 0.02).

More drop-outs due to side effects occurred in the LAAM group than methadone (two studies with 731 participants; RR 2.54, 95% CI 1.45–4.44, P = 0.001).

What this review adds to the current knowledge: Several studies on efficacy of LAAM maintenance were found. With respect to methadone, LAAM appears to be more effective at reducing heroin use. However, more LAAM patients than methadone ceased their allocated medication. More drop-outs due to side effects were observed in the LAAM group.

Main limitations: There was a significant heterogeneity between trials that assessed the outcome treatment cessation. Outcome reporting bias is another source of bias.

The future: The last assessment of this review was 2002. A subsequent randomised trial published in 2003 reported no significant differences between LAAM and methadone on retention in treatment, nor heroin use in 93 patients included.[2] Another trial that included 315 patients reported that LAAM and methadone patients did not differ on treatment retention, although LAAM patients were less likely to test positive for opiate use during treatment and at 26-week follow-up.[3]

128 **Drugs**

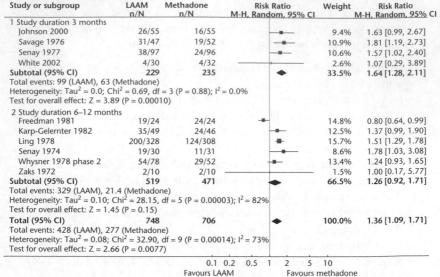

Review: LAAM maintenance vs methadone maintenance for heroin dependence
Comparison: 1 Treatment cessation
Outcome: 1 Cessation of allocated medication

Study or subgroup	LAAM n/N	Methadone n/N	Risk Ratio M-H, Random, 95% CI	Weight	Risk Ratio M-H, Random, 95% CI
1 Study duration 3 months					
Johnson 2000	26/55	16/55		9.4%	1.63 [0.99, 2.67]
Savage 1976	31/47	19/52		10.9%	1.81 [1.19, 2.73]
Senay 1977	38/97	24/96		10.6%	1.57 [1.02, 2.40]
White 2002	4/30	4/32		2.6%	1.07 [0.29, 3.89]
Subtotal (95% CI)	**229**	**235**		**33.5%**	**1.64 [1.28, 2.11]**
Total events: 99 (LAAM), 63 (Methadone)					
Heterogeneity: Tau^2 = 0.0; Chi^2 = 0.69, df = 3 (P = 0.88); I^2 = 0.0%					
Test for overall effect: Z = 3.89 (P = 0.00010)					
2 Study duration 6–12 months					
Freedman 1981	19/24	24/24		14.8%	0.80 [0.64, 0.99]
Karp-Gelernter 1982	35/49	24/46		12.5%	1.37 [0.99, 1.90]
Ling 1978	200/328	124/308		15.7%	1.51 [1.29, 1.78]
Senay 1974	19/30	11/31		8.6%	1.78 [1.03, 3.08]
Whysner 1978 phase 2	54/78	29/52		13.4%	1.24 [0.93, 1.65]
Zaks 1972	2/10	2/10		1.5%	1.00 [0.17, 5.77]
Subtotal (95% CI)	**519**	**471**		**66.5%**	**1.26 [0.92, 1.71]**
Total events: 329 (LAAM), 21.4 (Methadone)					
Heterogeneity: Tau^2 = 0.10; Chi^2 = 28.15, df = 5 (P = 0.00003); I^2 = 82%					
Test for overall effect: Z = 1.45 (P = 0.15)					
Total (95% CI)	**748**	**706**		**100.0%**	**1.36 [1.09, 1.71]**
Total events: 428 (LAAM), 277 (Methadone)					
Heterogeneity: Tau^2 = 0.08; Chi^2 = 32.90, df = 9 (P = 0.00014); I^2 = 73%					
Test for overall effect: Z = 2.66 (P = 0.0077)					

```
            0.1  0.2   0.5   1    2    5   10
            Favours LAAM        Favours methadone
```

Figure 48.1 LAAM versus methadone, outcome: cessation of allocated medication. Reproduced from Clark N, Lintzeris N, Gijsbers A, Whelan G, Dunlop A, Ritter A, *et al.* LAAM maintenance vs methadone maintenance for heroin dependence. Cochrane Database Syst Rev. 2002(2):CD002210, with permission from John Wiley & Sons Ltd. Copyright © 2002 The Cochrane Collaboration.

References

1 Clark N, Lintzeris N, Gijsbers A, Whelan G, Dunlop A, Ritter A, *et al.* LAAM maintenance vs methadone maintenance for heroin dependence. Cochrane Database Syst Rev. 2002(2):CD002210. Epub 2002/06/22.

2 Ritter AJ, Lintzeris N, Clark N, Kutin JJ, Bammer G, Panjari M. A randomised trial comparing levo-alpha acetylmethadol with methadone maintenance for patients in primary care settings in Australia. Addiction. 2003;98(11):1605–13. Epub 2003/11/18.

3 Longshore D, Annon J, Anglin MD, Rawson RA. Levo-alpha-acetylmethadol (LAAM) versus methadone: treatment retention and opiate use. Addiction. 2005;100(8):1131–9. Epub 2005/07/27.

Chapter 49 **Detoxification treatments for opiate-dependent adolescents**[1]

Review question: Is detoxification treatment alone or in combination with psychosocial intervention better than no intervention, other pharmacological intervention or psychosocial intervention in reducing substance use and improving health and social status?

What is known of this topic: Substance use among adolescents is a serious and growing problem. Managed withdrawal, or detoxification, is not in itself a treatment for dependence, but detoxification remains a required first step for many forms of longer term treatment. Different treatments have been tested in the management of opioid withdrawal in adults. However, little is known about the effectiveness of pharmacological detoxification among adolescents.

Summary: Evidence is limited to draw conclusions on the basis of two trials with limited sample size. None of these studies considered the efficacy of methadone.

Last assessment date: 17 October 2008

Objectives: To assess the effectiveness of detoxification treatment alone or in combination with psychosocial intervention compared to no intervention, other pharmacological intervention or psychosocial interventions on completion of treatment, reducing the use of substances and improving health and social status. *Primary outcomes*: Drop-outs, use of primary substance, acceptability of treatment and relapse at follow-up. *Other outcomes*: Engagement in further treatment, use of other substances, side effects, mortality, nonfatal overdose, criminal activity and social functioning.

Study population: Opiate-dependent adolescents (up to 18 years old).

Search strategy: Cochrane Central Register of Controlled Trials, MEDLINE, EMBASE, CINHAL (August 2008) and reference lists of articles.

Alcohol and Drug Misuse: A Cochrane Handbook, First Edition. Iosief Abraha and Cristina Cusi.
© 2012 John Wiley & Sons, Ltd. Published 2012 by John Wiley & Sons, Ltd.

Results: Two trials involving 190 participants were included.

- *Buprenorphine versus clonidine (one study):* There was no significant difference in drop-out from treatment (RR 0.45, 95% CI 0.20 −1.04, P = 0.063), although there was a trend in favour of buprenorphine. There was no significant difference in terms of duration and severity of signs and symptoms of withdrawal (WMD: 3.97, 95% CI −1.38 to 9.32). Adverse events were not reported.
- *Buprenorphine-naloxone maintenance versus buprenorphine detoxification (one study):* Outcomes such as drop-out rates (RR 2.67, 95% CI 1.85–3.86) and relapse at follow-up (RR 1.36, 95% CI 1.05–1.76) were in favour of maintenance treatment. Serious adverse events did not happen in both groups.

What this review adds to the current knowledge: Only two trials addressing the efficacy of detoxification treatment for opiate-dependent adolescents were identified. The two studies considered buprenorphine but not the efficacy of methadone that is still the most frequent drug utilised for the treatment of opioid withdrawal. Consequently, it is difficult to draw conclusions based on these two trials.

Main limitations: The sample size of the included studies was limited.

The future: Randomised trials comparing pharmacological detoxification (including methadone) versus psychosocial intervention and trials comparing pharmacological intervention and psychosocial intervention versus psychosocial intervention alone are warranted.

Reference

1 Minozzi S, Amato L, Davoli M. Detoxification treatments for opiate dependent adolescents. Cochrane Database Syst Rev. 2009(2):CD006749. Epub 2009/04/17.

Chapter 50 Maintenance treatments for opiate-dependent adolescents[1]

Review question: Is maintenance treatment alone or in combination with psychosocial intervention effective in reducing the use of substances and improving health and social status?

What is known of this topic: Pharmacological maintenance treatment is a necessary component of effective treatments for opioid dependence in adults. However, little is known as to whether maintenance therapy is effective in adolescents.

Summary: There is insufficient evidence to conclude that pharmacological treatment as a maintenance approach is effective in adolescents.

Last assessment date: 20 March 2008

Objectives: To assess the effectiveness of any maintenance treatment alone or in combination with psychosocial intervention compared to no intervention, pharmacological intervention or other psychosocial intervention on retaining adolescents in treatment, reducing the use of substances and improving health and social status. *Primary outcomes*: Drop-outs, use of primary substance and relapse at follow-up. *Other outcomes*: Use of other substances, side effects, mortality, nonfatal overdose, criminal activity and social functioning.

Study population: Opiate-dependent adolescents (up to 18 years old).

Search strategy: The Cochrane Drugs and Alcohol Group's trials register, MEDLINE, EMBASE and CINHAL (August 2008).

Results: Two trials involving 187 participants were included.
- *Buprenorphine–naloxone maintenance versus buprenorphine detoxification (one study)*: Maintenance treatment resulted better than control in terms

Alcohol and Drug Misuse: A Cochrane Handbook, First Edition. Iosief Abraha and Cristina Cusi.
© 2012 John Wiley & Sons, Ltd. Published 2012 by John Wiley & Sons, Ltd.

of drop-outs (RR 0.37, 95% CI 0.26–0.54) and results at follow-up (RR 0.73, 95% CI 0.57–0.95). There was no significant difference in terms of use of primary substance. No significant differences were observed in the secondary outcomes: adverse side effects, mortality and use of other substances (alcohol and marijuana).

- *LAAM versus methadone (one study)*: Data for all the primary outcomes were not reported.

What this review adds to the current knowledge: The presence of only two trials in the medical literature limits the indication of pharmacological treatment as a maintenance approach for adolescents.

Main limitations: The methodological quality and sample size of the studies were limited. Outcome reporting bias is another threat to the validity of the results.

The future: There is an urgent need of further randomised controlled trials comparing maintenance treatment with detoxification treatment or psychosocial treatment alone before realising studies which compare different pharmacological maintenance treatments. These studies should have long follow-up measuring the results of relapse after the end of treatment, and social functioning (integration at school or at work, and family relationship).

Reference

1 Amato L, Minozzi S, Davoli M, Vecchi S, Ferri MM, Mayet S. Psychosocial combined with agonist maintenance treatments versus agonist maintenance treatments alone for treatment of opioid dependence. Cochrane Database Syst Rev. 2008(4):CD004147.

Chapter 51 **Maintenance agonist treatments for opiate-dependent pregnant women**[1]

Review question: Is maintenance treatment alone or in combination with psychosocial intervention compared to no intervention (or other pharmacological intervention or psychosocial interventions) effective on child health status, neonatal mortality, retaining pregnant women in treatment and reducing use of substances?

What is known of this topic: Addicted women may continue to use opioids during pregnancy. Since heroin easily crosses the placenta, these women may experience a six-fold increase in maternal obstetric complications including low birth weight, toxaemia, third-trimester bleeding, malpresentation, puerperal morbidity, foetal distress and meconium aspiration. Newborns may experience narcotic withdrawal, postnatal growth deficiency, and increased neonatal mortality. Maintenance treatment with opioid antagonists may prevent the adverse effects on the foetus of repeated withdrawals.

Summary: There was no sufficient evidence to conclude for a specific treatment. Trials were too few and limited in size.

Last assessment date: 7 January 2008

Objectives: To assess the effectiveness of any maintenance treatment alone or in combination with psychosocial interventions compared to no intervention, other pharmacological interventions or psychosocial interventions. *Outcome for pregnant women*: Drop-out from treatment, use of primary substance and relapse at follow-up. *Outcome for the newborn*: Birth weight, APGAR score, Neonatal Abstinence Syndrome and prenatal and neonatal mortality. *Other outcomes*: Any problem of pregnancy, nicotine consumption, use of other substances, side effects for the mother and side effects for the child.

Study population: Opiate-dependent pregnant women of any age irrespective of duration of pregnancy.

Alcohol and Drug Misuse: A Cochrane Handbook, First Edition. Iosief Abraha and Cristina Cusi.
© 2012 John Wiley & Sons, Ltd. Published 2012 by John Wiley & Sons, Ltd.

Search strategy: The Cochrane Drugs and Alcohol Group's Register of Trials (June 2007), PubMed (1966–June 2007), CINAHL (1982–June 2007), reference lists of relevant papers, sources of on-going trials, conference proceedings and national focal points for drug research.

Results: Three trials with 96 participants were included.

For the woman

- *Methadone versus buprenorphine*: There was no statistical difference in terms of drop-out from treatment (two studies with 48 participants; RR 1.00, 95% CI 0.41–2.44) or use of primary substance of abuse (one study with 20 participants; RR 2.50, 95% CI 0.11–54.87).
- *Methadone versus slow morphine*: The results were in favour of oral slow morphine for the outcome use of substance (participants who used heroin in the third trimester) (one study with 20 participants; RR (fixed) 2.40, 95% CI 1.00 to 5.77). This result was not confirmed in the other trial.

For the child

- *Methadone versus buprenorphine*: Buprenorphine resulted better than methadone for the outcome birth weight (one study with 19 participants; WMD −530 gr, 95% CI −662 gr to −397 gr).

There were no statistical differences between the two treatments in terms of the outcomes: APGAR score, Neonatal Abstinence Syndrome, prenatal and neonatal mortality.

What this review adds to the current knowledge: Very few studies with limited participants were found. Although some results may be promising, the inherent limitations of the studies included limit the recommendation of maintenance agonist treatments for opiate-dependent pregnant women in clinical practice.

Main limitations: The trials were not adequately powered and were too few to detect any difference between the considered treatment.

The future: Well-designed and adequately powered randomised studies are necessary to sufficiently address these relevant issues. Future trials should compare different pharmacological maintenance treatments with longer follow-up periods.

Reference

1 Minozzi S, Amato L, Vecchi S, Davoli M. Maintenance agonist treatments for opiate dependent pregnant women. Cochrane Database Syst Rev. 2008(2):CD006318. Epub 2008/04/22.

Chapter 52 **Pharmacological treatment for depression during opioid agonist treatment for opioid dependence**[1]

Review question: Does treatment with antidepressant reduce the risk of depression in opioid-dependent subjects?

What is known of this topic: Depression is more common in people with substance use disorders than in the general population. Depression is also associated with an increased risk of suicide in opioid-dependent subjects.

Summary: There is insufficient evidence to indicate the use of antidepressants for the treatment of depressed opioid addicts.

Last assessment date: 19 July 2010

Objectives: To evaluate the efficacy and the acceptability of antidepressants for the treatment of depressed opioid dependents treated with opioid agonists. *Primary outcomes:* Drop-outs from the treatment, severity of depression measured with validated scales and acceptability of the treatment. *Other outcomes:* Use of primary substance, psychiatric symptoms and psychological distress diagnosed using standard criteria.

Study population: Opioid-dependent participants in treatment with a diagnosis of depression. The diagnosis of depression had to be carried out using standardised criteria, such as *Diagnostic and Statistical Manual of Mental Disorders* (DSM-IV-TR), *International Classification of Diseases* (ICD-10) or an equivalent, or by specialists.

Search strategy: PubMed, EMBASE, CINAHL (to October 2009), CENTRAL (The Cochrane Drug and Alcohol Group's Specialised Register), *The Cochrane Library* (Issue 4, 2009), main electronic sources of on-going trials and specific trial databases.

Alcohol and Drug Misuse: A Cochrane Handbook, First Edition. Iosief Abraha and Cristina Cusi.
© 2012 John Wiley & Sons, Ltd. Published 2012 by John Wiley & Sons, Ltd.

Results: Seven studies with 482 participants were included.

- Comparing antidepressant with placebo, no statistically significant results for dropouts: Selecting studies with low risk of bias, comprising 325 participants, results favour placebo (RR 1.40, CI 95% 1.00–1.96). For severity of depression, results from two studies, comprising 183 participants, favour antidepressants utilising the Clinical Global Impression Scale (RR 1.92, CI 95% 1.26–2.94), while another study of 95 participants, utilising the Hamilton Depression Rating Scale, did not find a statistically significant difference (RR 0.96, CI 95% 0.54–1.71). For adverse events, results favour placebo (four studies with 311 participants; RR 2.90, CI 95% 1.23–6.86). For substance use disorders (three studies with 211 participants), it was not possible to pool data because outcomes' measures were not comparable. Looking at singular studies, no statistically significant difference was seen.
- Comparing different classes of antidepressants, the results favour tricyclics for severity of depression (two studies with 183 participants; RR 1.92, CI 95% 1.26–2.94) and favour placebo for adverse events (two studies with 172 participants; RR 3.11, CI 95% 1.06–9.12).

What this review adds to the current knowledge: Although there were several studies published, the results were limited to support the use of antidepressants in opioid-dependent patients.

Main limitations: Small sample size and heterogeneity in terms of design, quality, characteristics of patients, tested medication, services and treatments delivered in the included studies.

The future: Randomised studies of high methodological quality and adequate sample size investigating relevant outcomes, safety issues and reporting data to allow comparison of results are needed.

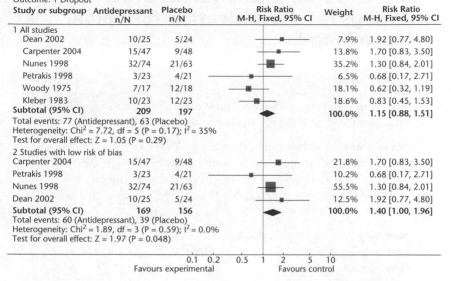

Review: Pharmacological treatment depression during opioid agonist treatment for opioid dependence
Comparison: 1 Antidepressants vs placebo accord to any definition
Outcome: 1 Dropout

Study or subgroup	Antidepressant n/N	Placebo n/N	Risk Ratio M-H, Fixed, 95% CI	Weight	Risk Ratio M-H, Fixed, 95% CI
1 All studies					
Dean 2002	10/25	5/24		7.9%	1.92 [0.77, 4.80]
Carpenter 2004	15/47	9/48		13.8%	1.70 [0.83, 3.50]
Nunes 1998	32/74	21/63		35.2%	1.30 [0.84, 2.01]
Petrakis 1998	3/23	4/21		6.5%	0.68 [0.17, 2.71]
Woody 1975	7/17	12/18		18.1%	0.62 [0.32, 1.19]
Kleber 1983	10/23	12/23		18.6%	0.83 [0.45, 1.53]
Subtotal (95% CI)	**209**	**197**		**100.0%**	**1.15 [0.88, 1.51]**
Total events: 77 (Antidepressant), 63 (Placebo)					
Heterogeneity: Chi² = 7.72, df = 5 (P = 0.17); I² = 35%					
Test for overall effect: Z = 1.05 (P = 0.29)					
2 Studies with low risk of bias					
Carpenter 2004	15/47	9/48		21.8%	1.70 [0.83, 3.50]
Petrakis 1998	3/23	4/21		10.2%	0.68 [0.17, 2.71]
Nunes 1998	32/74	21/63		55.5%	1.30 [0.84, 2.01]
Dean 2002	10/25	5/24		12.5%	1.92 [0.77, 4.80]
Subtotal (95% CI)	**169**	**156**		**100.0%**	**1.40 [1.00, 1.96]**
Total events: 60 (Antidepressant), 39 (Placebo)					
Heterogeneity: Chi² = 1.89, df = 3 (P = 0.59); I² = 0.0%					
Test for overall effect: Z = 1.97 (P = 0.048)					

0.1 0.2   0.5   1   2   5   10
Favours experimental   Favours control

Figure 52.1 Antidepressants versus placebo during opioid agonist treatment for opioid dependence, outcome: dropout. Reproduced from Pani PP, Vacca R, Trogu E, Amato L, Davoli M. Pharmacological treatment for depression during opioid agonist treatment for opioid dependence. Cochrane Database Syst Rev. 2010(9):CD008373, with permission from John Wiley & Sons Ltd. Copyright © 2010 The Cochrane Collaboration.

Reference

1 Pani PP, Vacca R, Trogu E, Amato L, Davoli M. Pharmacological treatment for depression during opioid agonist treatment for opioid dependence. Cochrane Database Syst Rev. 2010(9):CD008373.

Chapter 53 **Inpatient versus other settings for detoxification for opioid dependence**[1]

Review question: Is any inpatient opioid detoxification programme better than other time-limited detoxification programmes?

What is known of this topic: There are a complex range of variables that can influence the course and subjective severity of opioid withdrawal. There is a growing evidence for the effectiveness of a range of medically supported detoxification strategies, but little attention has been paid to the influence of the setting in which the process takes place.

Summary: There is no good available research to guide the clinician about the outcomes or cost-effectiveness of inpatient or outpatient approaches to opioid detoxification.

Last assessment date: 24 May 2008

Objectives: To evaluate the effectiveness of any inpatient opioid detoxification programme when compared with all other time-limited detoxification programmes. *Outcomes*: Level of completion of detoxification, the intensity and duration of withdrawal signs and symptoms, adverse effects, the level of engagement in further treatment post detoxification and the rates of lapse and relapse post detoxification.

Study population: Adult participants whose primary *International Classification of Diseases* (ICD-10) or *Diagnostic and Statistical Manual of Mental Disorders* (DSM-IV-TR) diagnosis is one of opioid dependence and who have undertaken a medically supported detoxification procedure.

Search strategy: *The Cochrane Library*, MEDLINE, EMBASE, PsycINFO, CINAHL (May 2008), Current Contents, Biological Abstracts, Science Citation Index and Social Sciences Index.

Alcohol and Drug Misuse: A Cochrane Handbook, First Edition. Iosief Abraha and Cristina Cusi.
© 2012 John Wiley & Sons, Ltd. Published 2012 by John Wiley & Sons, Ltd.

Results: Only one randomised study with 40 participants was included.

In the hospital detoxification group, seven out of 10 (70%) subjects were drug free at the end of the detoxification period, while in the outpatient detoxification 11 out of 30 (37%) participants were drug free at the end of the detoxification period. However, one-third of both groups were lost to follow-up. All hospital detoxification patients had returned to heroin use within 3 months of treatment. All but two of the outpatient detoxification patients had returned to heroin use within 2 months of treatment, and one of these was in prison.

What this review adds to the current knowledge: Only one published trial evaluated the effectiveness of an inpatient opioid detoxification programme. The results from this review do not add any substantial evidence to the current knowledge.

Main limitations: The single study included in this review was of limited methodological quality and inadequate sample size.

The future: Randomised trials of adequate sample size and methodological quality are warranted.

Reference

1 Day E, Ison J, Strang J. Inpatient versus other settings for detoxification for opioid dependence. Cochrane Database Syst Rev. 2005(2):CD004580. Epub 2005/04/23.

Chapter 54 **Psychotherapeutic interventions for cannabis use or dependence in outpatient settings**[1]

Review question: Are psychosocial interventions effective for cannabis use or dependence?

What is known of this topic: Cannabis use disorder is the most common illicit substance use disorder in the general population. Despite that, only a minority seek assistance from a health professional, but the demand for treatment is now increasing internationally. Trials of treatment have been published, but to our knowledge there is no published systematic review.

Summary: The heterogeneity of the treatment modalities and the limitation of the setting in which the studies were conducted hinder the possibility of drawing a sound recommendation.

Last assessment date: 20 April 2006

Objectives: To evaluate the efficacy of psychosocial interventions for cannabis use or dependence. *Primary outcomes*: Severity of substance use, self-reported use of cannabis and drop-out from treatment. *Other outcomes*: Frequency of other substance use and level of cannabis-related problems (e.g. medical problems, legal problems and social and family relations).

Study population: Participants who met diagnostic criteria for cannabis use or dependence, assessed by the *Diagnostic and Statistical Manual of Mental Disorders* (DSM-IV-TR) or *International Classification of Diseases* (ICD-10), and who sought treatment in outpatient settings.

Search strategy: Cochrane Central Register of Trials (2004), MEDLINE (August 2004), PsycINFO, CINAHL (October 2004), Toxibase (September 2004) and reference lists of articles.

Alcohol and Drug Misuse: A Cochrane Handbook, First Edition. Iosief Abraha and Cristina Cusi.
© 2012 John Wiley & Sons, Ltd. Published 2012 by John Wiley & Sons, Ltd.

Results: Six trials involving 1297 people were included.

Studies were not pooled in meta-analysis because of heterogeneity. The six included studies suggested that counselling approaches might have beneficial effects for the treatment of cannabis dependence. Group and individual sessions of cognitive-behavioural therapy (CBT) both had efficacy for the treatment of cannabis dependence and associated problems; CBT produced better outcomes than a brief intervention when CBT was delivered in individual sessions. Two studies suggested that adding voucher-based incentives may enhance retention in treatment when used in combination with other effective psychotherapeutic interventions. All included trials reported a statistically significant reduction in frequency of cannabis use and dependence symptoms. But other measures of problems related to cannabis use were not consistently different.

What this review adds to the current knowledge: The studies comparing different therapeutic modalities raise important questions about the duration, intensity and type of treatment. The generalisability of findings is also unknown because the studies have been conducted in a limited number of localities with heterogeneous samples of treatment seekers. However, the low abstinence rate indicated that cannabis dependence is not easily treated by psychotherapies in outpatient settings.

Main limitations: Heterogeneity among studies hindered the possibility of pooling results. The unclear allocation concealment in all studies is another source of concern.

The future: Response rates, particularly regarding abstinence from cannabis, leave much room for improvement. More multisite randomised trials with longer term outcomes should be conducted. Future studies should consider dismantling designs in which hypothesised active components of the interventions are offered individually or in specific combinations and are compared with appropriate attention–placebo interventions to control for number of sessions.

Reference

1 Denis C, Lavie E, Fatseas M, Auriacombe M. Psychotherapeutic interventions for cannabis abuse and/or dependence in outpatient settings. Cochrane Database Syst Rev. 2006(3):CD005336. Epub 2006/07/21.

Chapter 55 **Pharmacological interventions for benzodiazepine mono-dependence management in outpatient settings**[1]

Review question: Which pharmacological interventions are effective for benzodiazepine mono-dependence?

What is known of this topic: Since benzodiazepines are considered of high safety profile, the prevalence of their use is high worldwide. Benzodiazepines are effective as short-term treatments for some disorders; however, they are potentially addictive drugs. Evidence is needed about interventions for benzodiazepine dependence.

Summary: Gradual tapering was preferable to abrupt discontinuation. Carbamazepine appears to be an effective intervention for benzodiazepine gradual tapering discontinuation.

Last assessment date: 10 May 2006

Objectives: To evaluate the effectiveness of pharmacological interventions for outpatient management of benzodiazepine mono-dependence. *Primary outcomes*: Self-reported use of benzodiazepine with confirmation by urinalysis, retention in treatment, treatment compliance and severity of benzodiazepine withdrawal (assessed by validated questionnaire). *Other outcomes*: Self-reported use of other substances.

Study population: All adult patients who met criteria for benzodiazepine dependence were included regardless of gender and nationality. Exclusion criteria were current dependence on alcohol or any other drug (except nicotine).

Search strategy: The Cochrane Drugs and Alcohol Group's Register of Trials (October 2004), *The Cochrane Library* (Issue 4, 2004), MEDLINE, EMBASE, PsycINFO, CINAHL (October 2004), Pascal, Toxibase and reference lists of articles.

Results: Eight studies with 458 participants were included.

Study duration ranged from 4 to 14 weeks; some studies' follow-up after tapering ranged from 4 to 12 weeks. The presence of heterogeneity hindered

Alcohol and Drug Misuse: A Cochrane Handbook, First Edition. Iosief Abraha and Cristina Cusi.
© 2012 John Wiley & Sons, Ltd. Published 2012 by John Wiley & Sons, Ltd.

the possibility of performing meta-analyses. Following a gradual withdrawal process (over 10 weeks) appeared better than abrupt withdrawal. The number of drop-outs was lower with a gradual tapering process than with abrupt withdrawal, and the gradual procedure is judged more favourable by the participants. Short half-life benzodiazepine did not have higher withdrawal symptoms scores. Switching from short half-life benzodiazepine to long half-life benzodiazepine before gradual tapering withdrawal did not receive much support from this review. No benefits of propanolol, dothiepin, buspirone, progesterone or hydroxyzine were found for managing benzodiazepine withdrawal or improving benzodiazepine abstinence. Carbamazepine might have promise as an adjunctive medication for benzodiazepine withdrawal, particularly in patients receiving a daily dosage of 20 mg/d or more of diazepam (or equivalents).

> **What this review adds to the current knowledge:** All included studies showed that gradual tapering was preferable to abrupt discontinuation. However, the heterogeneity in the type of intervention and the type of population impedes the possibility of generalization. The results of this systematic review point to the potential value of carbamazepine to enhance retention and benzodiazepine-free status if coupled with benzodiazepine gradual tapering discontinuation. However, larger controlled studies are needed to confirm carbamazepine's potential benefit, to assess adverse effects and to identify when its clinical use might be the most indicated. Other treatment approaches to benzodiazepine discontinuation management should be explored (antidepressants and benzodiazepine receptor modulators).
>
> **Main limitations:** Significant heterogeneity was present.
>
> **The future:** Larger controlled studies are needed to confirm that switching from short half-life benzodiazepine to long half-life benzodiazepine before gradual tapering withdrawal did not have any impact regarding the intensity of the withdrawal symptoms.
>
> Larger controlled studies are needed to confirm carbamazepine's potential benefit, to assess adverse effects and to identify when its clinical use is indicated.
>
> Other suggested treatment approaches to benzodiazepine discontinuation management should be explored with Flumazenil, a benzodiazepine receptor antagonist that may be of benefit as it may up-regulate the benzodiazepine receptors; or antidepressants, on the basis of their ability to down-regulate monoaminergic receptors and to reduce both depression and anxiety levels, might also have benefits.

Reference

1 Denis C, Fatseas M, Lavie E, Auriacombe M. Pharmacological interventions for benzodiazepine mono-dependence management in outpatient settings. Cochrane Database Syst Rev. 2006(3):CD005194. Epub 2006/07/21.

Chapter 56 **Treatment for amphetamine dependence**[1]

Review question: What are the risks, benefits and costs of different treatment regimens (fluoxetine, amlodipine, imipramine and desipramine) for amphetamine dependence or use?

What is known of this topic: Amphetamines are psychostimulants of the phenethylamine class which produce increased wakefulness and increased activity levels, with a decrease in appetite. However, amphetamines are widely used because they produce euphoria. Dependence on amphetamines is more common than cocaine and heroin dependence combined. Interventions that help are needed for amphetamine dependence.

Summary: Fluoxetine, amlodipine, imipramine and desipramine have very limited benefits for amphetamine dependence and use.

Last assessment date: 16 Jul 2008

Objectives: To determine the risks, benefits and costs of a variety of treatments for amphetamine dependence or use. *Primary outcomes*: Rate of relapse, death and craving.

Study population: Participants with amphetamine dependence or use, diagnosed by any set of criteria.

Search strategy: The Cochrane Group on Drugs and Alcohol's specialised register of trials, MEDLINE, EMBASE, CINAHL, Cochrane Controlled Trials Register (January 2001) and references of obtained articles.

Results: Four studies with 173 participants were included.

Fluoxetine, amlodipine, imipramine and desipramine have been investigated in four randomised trials. In comparison to placebo, short-term

Alcohol and Drug Misuse: A Cochrane Handbook, First Edition. Iosief Abraha and Cristina Cusi.
© 2012 John Wiley & Sons, Ltd. Published 2012 by John Wiley & Sons, Ltd.

treatment of fluoxetine (40 mg/day) significantly decreased craving. In comparison to imipramine 10 mg/day, medium-term treatment of imipramine 150 mg/day significantly increased the duration of adherence to treatment. All four drugs had no benefits on a variety of outcomes, including amphetamine use.

What this review adds to the current knowledge: Fluoxetine, amlodipine, imipramine and desipramine were the interventions investigated for amphetamine dependence or use. Evidence from four RCTs is very limited. However, fluoxetine may decrease craving in short-term treatment, and imipramine may increase duration of adherence to treatment in medium-term treatment. Apart from these short-term benefits, no other advantages can be found.

Main limitations: Studies were of limited sample size, duration (maximum 8 weeks) and methodological quality.

The future: Although amphetamine dependence and use occur worldwide with a large number of people, very few controlled trials on this issue have been conducted. As trials using previous treatment show no promising results, other treatments, both biological and psychosocial, should be further investigated. In addition, the results of studies on the neurotoxicity of amphetamines are also crucial to design further studies for the evaluation of treatments for amphetamine dependence and use.

Reference

1 Srisurapanont M, Jarusuraisin N, Kittirattanapaiboon P. Treatment for amphetamine dependence and abuse. Cochrane Database Syst Rev. 2001(4):CD003022.

Chapter 57 **Treatment for amphetamine withdrawal**[1]

Review question: Which treatments are effective for amphetamine withdrawal?

What is known of this topic: Amphetamines are psychostimulants that are widely used because they produce euphoria and sometimes are used to treat depression. Use of amphetamines can lead to dependence similar to that of heroin or cocaine.

Summary: This review could not identify an effective treatment for amphetamine withdrawal.

Last assessment date: 8 February 2009

Objectives: To assess the effectiveness of pharmacological treatment alone or in combination with psychosocial treatment for amphetamine withdrawals on discontinuation rates, global state, withdrawal symptoms, craving and other outcomes.

Study population: Individuals with amphetamine withdrawal, diagnosed by any set of criteria.

Search strategy: MEDLINE, CINAHL, PsycINFO, CENTRAL (2008) and references of retrieved articles.

Results: Four randomised controlled trials involving 125 participants were included. Two studies found that amineptine significantly reduced discontinuation rates and improved overall clinical presentation, but did not reduce withdrawal symptoms or craving compared to placebo. The benefits of mirtazapine over placebo for reducing amphetamine withdrawal symptoms were not as clear. One study suggested that mirtazapine may reduce hyperarousal and anxiety symptoms associated with amphetamine withdrawal. Another study failed to find any benefit of mirtazapine over placebo on retention or on amphetamine withdrawal symptoms.

Alcohol and Drug Misuse: A Cochrane Handbook, First Edition. Iosief Abraha and Cristina Cusi.
© 2012 John Wiley & Sons, Ltd. Published 2012 by John Wiley & Sons, Ltd.

What this review adds to the current knowledge: The results of this review suggest that amineptine has some limited benefits in increasing adherence to treatment and improving general condition but has no direct benefit on specific amphetamine withdrawal symptoms or craving. Amineptine has been, however, withdrawn from the market. Mirtazapine did not have any effect on adherence to treatment, general condition, amphetamine withdrawal symptoms or cravings. However, this result was based on the data of one study. In conclusion, there are currently no available medications that have been demonstrated to be effective in the treatment of amphetamine withdrawal.

Main limitations: Although the studies were of low risk of bias, they were of limited sample size.

The future: There are few medications that have been evaluated. Amphetamine withdrawal seems a reasonable target for developing a medication to aid individuals in instilling amphetamine abstinence. Chronic amphetamine users seeking treatment must successfully resolve amphetamine withdrawal when establishing sustained abstinence from the drug. It remains unknown whether improved outcomes in successfully resolving amphetamine withdrawal would also correspond with longer term abstinence outcomes.

There is good reason to consider medications for amphetamine withdrawal that demonstrate propensities to increase central dopamine, norepinephrine and/or serotonin activities. Naturalistic studies of amphetamine withdrawal symptoms and courses are also crucial for the development of study designs appropriate for further treatment studies of amphetamine withdrawal.

Reference

1 Shoptaw SJ, Kao U, Heinzerling K, Ling W. Treatment for amphetamine withdrawal. Cochrane Database Syst Rev. 2009(2):CD003021. Epub 2009/04/17.

Chapter 58 **Treatment for amphetamine psychosis**[1]

Review question: What are the benefits and risks of treatments such as olanzapine and haloperidol used for amphetamine psychosis?

What is known of this topic: Amphetamine users may develop psychotic symptoms including paranoid and persecutory delusions as well as auditory and visual hallucinations in the presence of extreme agitation. In other instances, frequent amphetamine users may report psychotic symptoms that are subclinical and that do not require high-intensity intervention. It has been suggested that dopamine antagonists, such as chlorpromazine, haloperidol and thioridazine, are effective for the treatment of amphetamine psychosis.

Summary: Olanzapine and haloperidol at clinically relevant doses had effective results in resolving psychotic symptoms. The small study sample of the one trial published, however, makes it difficult to make this recommendation with confidence.

Last assessment date: 21 January 2009

Objectives: To search and determine risks, benefits and costs of available treatments for amphetamine psychosis. *Outcomes*: The number of people who respond to treatment, incidence of extrapyramidal side effects, discontinuation rate, death, global status, side effects, patient satisfaction, health status or health-related quality of life and economic outcomes.

Study population: People with amphetamine psychosis, diagnosed by any set of criteria.

Search strategy: MEDLINE, EMBASE, CINAHL, PsycINFO (2007), *The Cochrane Library* (Issue 1, 2008) and references of retrieved articles.

Alcohol and Drug Misuse: A Cochrane Handbook, First Edition. Iosief Abraha and Cristina Cusi.
© 2012 John Wiley & Sons, Ltd. Published 2012 by John Wiley & Sons, Ltd.

Results: One trial with 58 participants was included. The results show that both olanzapine and haloperidol at 7.5 mg/day and 7.8 mg/day were efficacious in resolving psychotic symptoms, with the olanzapine condition showing significantly greater safety and tolerability than the haloperidol control as measured by frequency and severity of extrapyramidal symptoms.

What this review adds to the current knowledge: The evidence derives from only one trial that showed that both olanzapine and haloperidol, at clinically relevant doses, can be effective in treating patients with amphetamine psychosis. However, the haloperidol condition experienced significantly more extrapyramidal side effects compared to olanzapine.

Main limitations: The evidence of the treatment for amphetamine psychosis is limited mainly due to the small sample size of the only trial published in the literature.

The future: Findings from one trial indicate that use of antipsychotic medications effectively resolves symptoms of acute amphetamine psychosis. This raises significant clinical questions regarding the clinical benefit to continued or episodic regimens of antipsychotic medications following resolution of acute amphetamine psychosis. High-quality randomised trials of conventional antipsychotics, newer antipsychotics and benzodiazepines for treating acute psychosis are needed.

Reference

1 Shoptaw SJ, Kao U, Ling W. Treatment for amphetamine psychosis. Cochrane Database Syst Rev. 2009(1):CD003026. Epub 2009/01/23.

Chapter 59 **Treatment for methaqualone dependence in adults**[1]

Review question: Are pharmacological or behavioural interventions effective for subjects affected by methaqualone dependence in comparison with no treatment?

What is known of this topic: Methaqualone is a potent quinazoline (a class of sedative-hypnotics) that has a high potential for misuse. Use of methaqualone (e.g. Quaalude or Mandrax) has waned in Western countries since the mid- to late 1980s; however, the practice of smoking methaqualone is a serious public health problem in Africa and India. Effective treatment for methaqualone dependence is needed.

Summary: No randomised clinical trials (RCTs) that evaluated treatment to reduce methaqualone use have been conducted.

Last assessment date: 30 September 2010

Objectives: To compare the effectiveness of any type of pharmacological or behavioural treatment administered in either an inpatient or outpatient setting compared with a placebo, no treatment or a waiting list, or with another form of treatment administered in either an inpatient or outpatient setting. *Primary outcomes:* Abstinence from methaqualone at 3 months and completion of treatment as measured. *Other outcomes:* Quality of life.

Study population: Voluntary, consenting adults who are dependent (according to *Diagnostic and Statistical Manual of Mental Disorders* (DSM-IV-TR) criteria) on methaqualone that was either orally ingested or smoked in combination with cannabis and tobacco.

Search strategy: The Cochrane Drugs and Alcohol Group's Register of Trials (February 2004), *The Cochrane Library* (Issue 2, 2004), MEDLINE, PsycINFO (February 2004), relevant conference proceedings and reference lists of relevant articles.

Alcohol and Drug Misuse: A Cochrane Handbook, First Edition. Iosief Abraha and Cristina Cusi.
© 2012 John Wiley & Sons, Ltd. Published 2012 by John Wiley & Sons, Ltd.

Results: No RCTs or quasi-RCTs were found that met the inclusion criteria.

> **What this review adds to the current knowledge:** Despite an extensive search of electronic databases, the internet and relevant conferences and contact with experts in the field, this review identified no RCTs of the effectiveness of treatment for methaqualone dependence and/or use. Currently no evidence exists for using one type of treatment over another.
>
> **Main limitations:** No studies were included.
>
> **The future:** The effectiveness of inpatient versus outpatient treatment, psychosocial treatment versus no treatment and pharmacological treatments versus placebo for methaqualone use or dependence has yet to be established.

Reference

1 McCarthy G, Myers B, Siegfried N. Treatment for methaqualone dependence in adults. Cochrane Database Syst Rev. 2005(2):CD004146. Epub 2005/04/23.

Index

Note: Page numbers in *italics* refer to Figures.

Alcohol and Drug Misuse: A Cochrane Handbook, First Edition. Iosief Abraha and
Cristina Cusi.
© 2012 John Wiley & Sons, Ltd. Published 2012 by John Wiley & Sons, Ltd.